COLUMBIA REVIEW

MCAT
Verbal Reasoning
Powerbuilder

COLUMBIA REVIEW

MCAT Verbal Reasoning Powerbuilder

Stephen D. Bresnick, M.D.

Attending Surgeon
Division of Plastic Surgery
University of Southern California
School of Medicine
Los Angeles, California
Co-Director, Columbia Review
San Francisco, California

William H. Bresnick, M.D.

Attending Physician and Clinical Instructor
San Francisco General Hospital
University of California, San Francisco,
School of Medicine
Co-Director, Columbia Review
San Francisco, California

SANS TACHE

Williams & Wilkins
A WAVERLY COMPANY

BALTIMORE • PHILADELPHIA • LONDON • PARIS • BANGKOK
BUENOS AIRES • HONG KONG • MUNICH • SYDNEY • TOKYO • WROCLAW

Editor: Elizabeth A. Nieginski
Manager, Development Editing: Julie Scardiglia
Managing Editor: Darrin Kiessling
Marketing Manager: Chris Brenchley
Copy Editor: Alethea Elkins
Development Editor: Beth Goldner
Production Coordinator: Felecia R. Weber
Designer: Nancy Hagan-Abbott
Illustration Planner: Felecia R. Weber
Cover Designer: Nancy Hagan-Abbott
Typesetter: Port City Press, Inc.
Printer: Port City Press, Inc.
Digitized Illustrations: Port City Press, Inc.
Binder: Port City Press, Inc.

351 West Camden Street
Baltimore, Maryland 21201-2436 USA

Rose Tree Corporate Center
1400 North Providence Road
Building II, Suite 5025
Media, Pennsylvania 19063-2043 USA

Printed in the United States of America

First Edition

Library of Congress Cataloging-in-Publication Data
Bresnick, Stephen D.
Columbia Review MCAT verbal reasoning powerbuilder / Stephen D. Bresnick. — 1st ed.
p. cm.
ISBN 0-683-30073-3
1. Medical colleges—United States—Entrance examinations—Study guides. 2. Reading comprehension—Problems, exercises, etc. 3. Reasoning—Problems, exercises, etc. I. Columbia Review, Inc. II. Title. III. Title: MCAT verbal reasoning powerbuilder
[DNLM: 1. Medicine—examination questions. 2. Verbal Learning—examination questions. 3. Reading—examination questions. W 18.2
B842ca 1997]
R838.5.B745 1997
610'.76—dc21
DNLM/DLC
for Library of Congress 97-3577
CIP

To purchase additional copies of this book, call our customer service department at **(800) 638-0672** or fax orders to **(800) 447-8438.** For other book services, including chapter reprints and large quantity sales, ask for the Special Sales department.

Canadian customers should call **(800) 665-1148** or fax **(800) 665-0103.** For all other calls originating outside of the United States, please call **(410) 528-4223** or fax us at **(410) 528-8550.**

Visit Williams & Wilkins on the Internet: **http://www.wwilkins.com** or contact our customer service department at **custserv@wwilkins.com.** Williams & Wilkins customer service representatives are available from 8:30 am to 6:00 pm, EST, Monday through Friday, for telephone access.

97 98 99 00
1 2 3 4 5 6 7 8 9 10

DEDICATION

The authors dedicate this book to Mrs. Irene Bresnick, for her 40 years of devotion to English teaching and education, and her commitment to excellence.

CONTENTS

Preface *ix*

Acknowledgments *xi*

CHAPTER 1 An Introduction to the MCAT Verbal Reasoning Section *1*

CHAPTER 2 Strategies for Verbal Reasoning Success *7*

CHAPTER 3 Reading Speed and Habits *15*

CHAPTER 4 Context and Meaning: Improving Comprehension of MCAT Passages *33*

CHAPTER 5 Using Key Words to Read and Comprehend *45*

CHAPTER 6 Skimming, Scanning, and Marking Text *55*

CHAPTER 7 Qualifiers and Distractors *69*

CHAPTER 8 Eye and Hand Movements for Faster, More Effective Reading *77*

CHAPTER 9 Speed-Reading Scientific and Other Specialized Material *91*

CHAPTER 10 Review Exercises and Practice Verbal Reasoning Passages *101*

CHAPTER 11 Verbal Reasoning Practice Tests *117*

Interpreting Scores on the Verbal Reasoning Practice Tests *219*

Reading Speed Goal Sheet *221*

Appendix *223*

PREFACE

Many medical school admissions committees believe that the Verbal Reasoning test is the most important section of the MCAT. The Verbal Reasoning test is challenging, difficult to finish, and stressful. Because the Verbal Reasoning test is the first section of the MCAT, it is important to do well, setting the tone for the rest of the exam.

Although the Verbal Reasoning section is important to MCAT success, many students do not take it seriously. Students often take for granted that they will do well; however, the results of student performance on the Verbal Reasoning section show that over 50% of students will score at the mean or below. Low or mediocre Verbal Reasoning scores often play an important role in determining whether or not a student is accepted to medical school.

Reading ability is a skill that a student develops over his or her lifetime. Improvement can only come when a student identifies his or her reading weaknesses and comprehension problems and works to correct those problems. To help students identify and address areas in which their reading may improve, Columbia Review has developed a new, intensive MCAT Verbal Reasoning program.

The *Columbia Review MCAT Verbal Reasoning Powerbuilder* is the first book solely dedicated to helping you improve your MCAT Verbal Reasoning scores. It has been specially designed to help enhance your reading abilities and give you new strategies for MCAT Verbal Reasoning success. This book emphasizes **speed reading and comprehension strategies**, **prescriptive teaching**, and **exercises** through features such as:

- Strategic discussions on how to take the Verbal Reasoning test
- Practice passages throughout the chapters
- Exercises and drills to improve reading
- Three full-length MCAT Verbal Reasoning tests
- Answers and explanations to all questions
- A vocabulary development program

Take advantage of this unique opportunity to simultaneously improve your MCAT scores and your reading ability!

ACKNOWLEDGMENTS

The authors wish to thank Jennifer Jackson, Diane Scott, and Dr. Steven Lincoln for their valuable contributions. In addition, many thanks to the staff of Williams & Wilkins for their dedication in creating a unique, high-quality book for MCAT Verbal Reasoning. We especially thank Beth Goldner, Elizabeth Nieginski, Kevin Thibodeau, and Tim Satterfield for their expertise and assistance with this important project.

Chapter 1

An Introduction to the MCAT Verbal Reasoning Section

Importance

Why is Verbal Reasoning So Important?

The Verbal Reasoning test may be the most important section of the MCAT because some medical schools think that Verbal Reasoning performance strongly correlates with medical school success. This surprises some premedical students who believe that the Physical or Biological sciences sections are more important than Verbal Reasoning.

Medical schools place a strong emphasis on the verbal section for several reasons. First, studies have shown that Verbal Reasoning success may correlate with higher scores on the United States Medical Licensing Exams (National Board Exams). Second, ineffective reading skills hinder medical students from keeping up with the enormous amount of reading and study required in medical school. Poor Verbal Reasoning scores also might indicate problems with students' study and communication skills. Many medical schools combine Verbal Reasoning scores in an admission formula to calculate point totals for applicants. A low Verbal Reasoning score means fewer admission points, which decreases the applicant's chances of gaining admission to medical school! For more details, please refer to *Columbia Review Intensive Preparation for the MCAT*.

Most students agree that the Verbal Reasoning test is the most difficult section of the MCAT. The test is graded on a curve, and because many premedical students are strong readers, the competition is tough.

Preparing for the MCAT

How Will This Book Help Me?

The *MCAT Verbal Reasoning Powerbuilder* emphasizes strategies and techniques to maximize your reading ability. Many important speed-reading and reading comprehension strategies are presented. Try each technique, working through the practice passages in the Powerbuilder, and you will quickly see which techniques and strategies work best for you. Remember to keep an open mind! Push yourself to try some new things. The purpose of the Powerbuilder is not to revolutionize your reading techniques shortly before the MCAT. **The goal is to build on your existing skills by adding tools to improve your speed and comprehension.** Thousands of premedical students have worked through the *MCAT Verbal Reasoning Powerbuilder* and found it incredibly useful in improving their scores.

We suggest that you work carefully and methodically through the Powerbuilder. Complete all the sample passages and exercises. When you have worked through these passages, obtain as many additional Verbal Reasoning passages as you can. Three additional full-length practice Verbal Reasoning tests can be found in *Columbia Review Intensive Preparation for the MCAT* (check your college bookstore or call

Williams & Wilkins at 1-800-638-0672 to order). Many more additional passages are available in the Columbia Review Home Study Course (call 1-800-300-7737 for information). The key to success is practice, practice, practice!

What Should I Do If English is My Second Language and/or I am a Remedial Reader?

If you are reading below the average level for a college student, you might need some help. This type of problem must be worked on well before taking the MCAT. As you know, reading ability is acquired during a lifetime, and significant reading problems are difficult to overcome in a short amount of time. You will need at least a year before the MCAT to improve your reading skills. In addition to working through this book, consider these options:

- Check with your local college or university to see if speed-reading and reading comprehension courses are available. Choose a course that emphasizes both speed and comprehension.
- Read several hours a day.
- If it is early in your college career, you can take reading-based humanities courses to help improve your verbal abilities.
- Consider consulting with your premedical advisor to decide which plan works best for you.

If you think that you are a remedial reader, have a reading specialist evaluate you. If your reading difficulties stem from a learning disability or a visual disturbance, it is possible to get extra time on the MCAT. You need documentation from a licensed health professional to apply for a special circumstance MCAT sitting. Up to double the usual time may be given to a student with a documented learning or visual disability. Do not be embarrassed by a diagnosed disability. This will not keep you from medical school. It just means that you need more time allocated for testing. Contact the American Association of Medical Colleges (AAMC) in Washington, DC for details.

Format

Before starting the *MCAT Verbal Reasoning Powerbuilder,* you must understand what the Verbal Reasoning test is all about. Take a minute to glance at one of the three full-length practice Verbal Reasoning tests in the back of this book. You will see that each test is approximately 16–20 pages and arranged into passages. Make a mental picture of what you see.

How is the Verbal Reasoning Section of the MCAT Laid Out? (Table 1-1)

Many Verbal Reasoning passages are complex and cover subjects with which you are not familiar. Recent MCAT passages have emphasized philosophy, art, history, humanities, and social sciences.

Table 1-1. MCAT Verbal Reasoning Test

Number of passages	9
Total time	85 minutes
Average passage length	500–600 words
Number of questions per passage	6–10
Total number of questions	65

Finishing the test on time is a common problem. This is true particularly if English is not a student's first language. As you move through the test, the passages become progressively harder and more complex. Even students who are strong readers complain that the Verbal Reasoning section is too long to finish in the given time. If you are a slow reader or English is your second language, **expect the length of this test to be a potential problem.** Frequently, students who finish the Verbal Reasoning test do so at the expense of carelessness. To overcome this timing problem, you must work hard to improve your speed and comprehension.

The difficulty levels of the questions that follow a passage are averaged, and the resulting average difficulty level is assigned to that set of questions. As a whole, the Verbal Reasoning test often progresses from least to most difficult, but individual passages contain both easy and more difficult questions.

Content

Topics Covered

The passages in the Verbal Reasoning section come from a variety of disciplines in the social sciences, humanities, and natural sciences (fields not covered in the Biological or Physical sciences). The following **three main disciplines** appear on the exam.

1. **Social sciences:** anthropology, archaeology, business, economics, law, government, history, political science, psychology, and sociology
2. **Humanities:** architecture, art, art history, dance, ethics, literary criticism, music, philosophy, religion, and theater
3. **Natural sciences:** astronomy, botany, computer science, ecology, geology, meteorology, natural history, and technology

Social science and humanities passages are difficult for most premedical students. These passages often contain arguments, subtle clues, inferences, opinions, and assertions. Students must sort through these elements to answer the questions. The goal of the social science and humanities passages is to assess your ability to analyze literature that is nonscientific and complex.

Of the three main disciplines, most students find that the natural science passages are easiest because many premedical students are science majors and feel comfortable with the content. These passages generally do not cover topics taught in introductory science courses. The goal of the natural science passages is to assess your ability to understand large amounts of new information, technical descriptions, and conceptual details.

As a whole, the passages discuss many different fields. However, you are not expected to have knowledge in all of these areas. The verbal section of the exam is designed to test your ability to read and comprehend text, then evaluate and apply the information. All the information needed to answer the questions appears in the passages.

MCAT Report: Recent Verbal Reasoning Passage Topics

A good way to get a sense of what to expect on the Verbal Reasoning test is to see what recent tests have been like. The following list of passage topics has been compiled to show you how the test makers mix passage topics to include the social sciences, humanities, and the natural sciences. Recent passage topics on the MCAT include:

- Greek art
- Geological formation of the Himalayas

- Welfare reform
- Authenticity of Roman statues
- Republicans
- An analysis of the book *Animal Farm*
- World War I poets
- Recent views on the Irish potato famine
- The writing of plays and stories
- Taxes during the American Revolution
- The need to teach ethics
- Platonic versus Aristotelian theater
- Galileo's vindication of Copernicus
- Women authors in the Victorian era
- French philosophers
- The effects of artificial light on circadian rhythms
- The significance of yeast
- Experimental psychology

Types of Writing

There are **three broad categories** of writing that appear on the exam.

1. **Narrative.** This is a record of events that happened in a given time period. A narrative passage usually tells a story.
2. **Expository/Informative.** This type of passage provides information about a subject.
3. **Argument.** In this type of passage, the author presents and defends a position on a controversial topic. An argument may contain inductive and/or deductive reasoning, and points in the argument can be explicitly or implicitly stated by the author.

Skills Tested

The Verbal Reasoning section of the MCAT is designed to test your reading comprehension and reasoning skills. The authors of the test have written questions to assess your abilities in four areas: **comprehension, evaluation, application,** and **incorporation of new information.**

Comprehension

Comprehension skills are measured by **questions that address what the writer said.** Questions may ask about information given in the passage, the position taken by the writer, evidence used to support that position, assumptions made by the writer, or conclusions that are or could be made. According to the *MCAT Student Manual,* the student uses the following skills in the comprehension category:

1. Identify the central concern or thesis of the passage.
2. Identify the reasons or evidence offered to support a thesis.
3. Identify background knowledge contained in the passage or question that is relevant to a particular interpretation.
4. Determine, from context, the meaning of significant terminology or vocabulary used in the passage.
5. Recognize an accurate paraphrase of complex information presented in the passage.
6. Identify comparative relationships among ideas or pieces of information in the passage.

7. Identify stated or unstated assumptions in the passage.
8. Recognize appropriate questions of clarification.

Evaluation

Evaluation skills test your ability to make a **judgment about an author's argument.** A writer uses inductive and/or deductive reasoning as evidence to support the position being argued. Evaluation questions ask you to consider the reliability, credibility, relevance, sufficiency, or accuracy of the evidence used by the writer. An evaluation question may have you determine the validity of the argument. The following skills are tested in the evaluation category:

1. Judge the soundness of an argument or a step of reasoning presented in the passage.
2. Judge the credibility of a source.
3. Judge if a conclusion follows necessarily from the reasons given in the passage.
4. Appraise the strength of the evidence for a generalization, conclusion, or claim.
5. Distinguish between supported and unsupported claims.
6. Judge the relevance of information to an argument or claim.

Application

Application questions expect you to **go beyond the author's message** to solve a related problem, interpret a hypothetical situation, identify a probable cause of an event, or identify a general theory or model that is applicable. The following skills are used to complete the application category:

1. Predict a result based on passage content and specific facts about a hypothetical situation.
2. Use given information to solve a specified problem.
3. Identify the probable cause of a particular event or result based on information presented.
4. Determine the implications of conclusions or results for real-world situations.
5. Recognize the scope of application of hypotheses, explanations, and conclusions.
6. Identify a general theory or model based on given information.

Incorporation of New Information

In this category, the question provides additional information. You need to **reconsider the author's argument** in light of this new information. You are expected to think beyond what the author presented as you answer these questions. The following skills are used in the incorporation of new information category:

1. Judge the bearing of new evidence on conclusions presented in the passage.
2. Recognize methods or results that would challenge hypotheses, models, or theories given in the passage.
3. Determine how a conclusion from the passage can be modified to be made consistent with additional information.
4. Recognize plausible alternative hypotheses or solutions.

Verbal Reasoning Questions

Categories of Questions

Six main categories of questions appear on the MCAT Verbal Reasoning section.

1. **Fact** questions test your comprehension of material explicitly stated in the passage.

2. **Inference** questions test your ability to comprehend the information given, draw conclusions about this information, and answer questions using these conclusions.
3. **Main idea** questions ask you to identify the central theme of the passage.
4. **Tone** questions ask you to sense the attitude of the passage.
5. **Application** questions ask you to take a concept presented in the passage and apply it to a new situation.
6. **Structure** questions ask you about the flow of information in the passage.

Types of Questions

There are only two major types of questions:

Multiple Choice

Multiple choice questions can test any of the four skills just discussed in Skills Tested. There will be four choices following each question (A–D). The correct answer is the **best** choice, which is tricky because there may be more than one correct statement among the four choices. Always remember to choose the *best* correct statement.

Extended Multiple Choice

This type of question also can test any of the four skills. In this format, three statements usually follow the question, I, II, and III. You choose which of those statements is correct and then choose the right answer. Again, there will be four choices (A–D) following each question. For example, choice A in the answer key might be that "I and II only" are true, choice B might say "I only," choice C might say "II and III only," and choice D might read "I, II, and III" are true.

Now that you are familiar with the importance and structure of the Verbal Reasoning test, you are ready to begin working on your reading skills. The next chapter will help determine your current reading speed, identify some common reading problems, and introduce some important strategies for the Verbal Reasoning test.

Chapter 2

Strategies for Verbal Reasoning Success

This chapter reviews some basic techniques and provides a brief introduction to important strategies for succeeding on the MCAT Verbal Reasoning section. These strategies and others are discussed in more detail later in this book. We recommend working through this chapter now and reviewing it several times as you work through this book. Some of the strategies are best understood when you have had a chance to work on Verbal Reasoning passages.

Approaching the Test

Before you begin working on practice Verbal Reasoning passages, it is important for you to have a mental game plan for how to approach the test. These basic strategies are important to think about and master (Table 2-1).

Basic Strategies

You must be totally motivated to do well on the Verbal Reasoning section. Make it a priority to work through this book and practice verbal passages.

You must concentrate on your reading and not let any distractions affect you. Do not let your mind wander as you read. One problem you will face when reading MCAT passages is **maintaining your concentration.** Many of the passages are dry and uninteresting, so it is natural for your concentration to wander. Have you ever had your eyes move down a column of reading material while your mind was elsewhere? You must **concentrate deeply** and completely when reading MCAT Verbal Reasoning passages.

You should have a planned approach to the test. There are two basic ways to approach the Verbal Reasoning passages. Most students prefer the first technique, in which question stems are skimmed before the passage is read. Other students find this technique somewhat distracting and prefer to start reading the passage before reading questions. The best way to see which approach works best for you is to try them both on some of the practice reading comprehension passages found in this book.

Table 2-1. Strategies for Approaching the Test

Be motivated
Concentrate
Use a planned approach
Do not read emotionally
Use first impressions
Determine order of passages
Practice timing

Approach 1: Skim Question Stems, Read Passage, Then Carefully Read Questions

1. Read through the questions before reading the passage and underline stems, key phrases, main ideas, and important words (e.g., except, only, always). A **question stem** is the part of the question that asks you a specific thing or gives you a task to perform. Make a mental picture of what the author is stressing or asking about. Spend no more than 15–20 seconds reading the question stems.
2. Read the passage and look for the key words and stems from the questions and mark (underline, circle, note in margins) the passage accordingly.
3. Reread each question carefully and look back at the passage. The marks you made will connect the question to the appropriate part of the passage.

Consider trying this question-stem reading technique. It is not necessary to read the answer choices. The purpose of question-stem reading is to preview what will be important in the passage. Practice this strategy. Question-stem previewing is a legal and ethical way to already know the questions before even reading the passage! Make sure that you spend only 15–20 seconds total on question-stem previewing. You only need to skim the question stems to learn which topics will be discussed.

This strategy helps many students with the Verbal Reasoning test, yet some other students find that question-stem previewing distracts them. Try this strategy for yourself to see if it helps. If you find question-stem previewing too distracting, consider using Approach 2.

Approach 2: Skim Topic Sentences, Read Passage, Then Answer Questions

1. Start by skimming the topic sentences of each paragraph to preview the passage. This helps you form a mental picture of the flow and main idea of the passage.
2. Read the passage, underlining or circling key ideas and main points, and making brief notes summarizing material in the margins. Feel free to read at a variable speed. Speed up if you understand or are familiar with the material. Slow down if the discussion gets complicated.
3. Next, read the questions and refer back to your highlights and margin notes to answer the questions.

Whichever method you choose, you should practice reading selections and answering questions as much as possible. Practice will hone your comprehension skills and make your reading more time efficient.

Do not get emotionally involved. Read from a distance. Frequently MCAT passages will offer discussion on an issue or event. These passages may present a point of view. Even if you disagree with the points or opinions expressed, try to remain neutral and only answer questions based on the facts or opinions evident in the passage.

Always use common sense, and go with your first impression. Although this advice seems obvious, many students lose sight of basic common sense under the stress of the MCAT. If you seem to understand the passage, an answer choice that appears the most logical is probably correct. Your **first logical impression** is often the correct answer. Therefore, do not change your answer unless you have a good reason.

You do not have to complete the passages in order! Most students find it easiest to work through the passages in order. This minimizes disorganization. However, if you come across a passage that is very difficult for you, it may be strategic to skip it and move on to an easier passage. If you are going to skip around, **work first on passages containing the most questions.** Remember, your score is determined by the number of questions you answer correctly.

Get your timing down! Timing is a key strategy. **You are severely punished for not finishing the Verbal Reasoning test.** There is no penalty for guessing, so you should answer every question on the test. However, randomly guessing on questions that you do not have time to read and evaluate means that you will only get approximately 25% of these correct. Because the Verbal Reasoning section is so competitive, guessing on many questions means you probably will not do well. Students often do not finish this section because they mismanage their time. We do not want this to happen to you! Here are some simple strategies to get your timing in order:

1. **Start by looking at the last passage in the Verbal Reasoning test.** Because each passage is numbered, the number of the last passage tells you how many total passages are on the exam. For example, if the last passage is number 9, there are nine passages on the test. Most recently, there have been nine passages on this section. Several years ago, there were 10 passages.
2. **Next, divide the number of passages into the total time allotted for the section.** You will be given 85 minutes total. Thus, divide 9 into 85 minutes. This gives approximately 9 minutes per passage with roughly 4 minutes remaining to either check your work or go back to difficult questions.
3. **Every three passages, you must check the time.** If by the end of the third passage you are more than 27 minutes (3 x 9 min/passage) into the test, you are working too slowly. Adjust your pace and speed up!

If you follow this simple approach, you will have the best chance of finishing the test. Because many of the other students mismanage their time and do not finish, this will give you an advantage.

Reading the Passages (Table 2-2)

Be an active reader. Think as you read! Ask yourself questions about what you are reading. What is the main idea? Why is the author discussing a particular topic? What is the tone? What is emphasized in the passage? On the MCAT, never be a passive reader. If you are not thinking about what you are reading, you will have more difficulty with comprehension.

Make a mental map of the passage. As you read the passage, create a mental picture of its layout. Think about how the author develops the ideas. Make a few notes in the margin next to each paragraph identifying the basic idea or theme of the paragraph. The mental map and notes that you make will help you rapidly find answers to the questions that follow the passage.

Focus on the topic sentences of the paragraphs. The main idea and important points in a passage generally are provided in the **first** and **last** sentences of each paragraph. Pay special attention to the topic sentences of the paragraphs as you read.

Mark the text as you read, noting key words, phrases, and ideas. You are encouraged to write in the test booklet. Use the margins for short notations and comments. Circling and underlining are also useful. If you do not mark up the Verbal Reasoning test, you are making a big mistake! Specific marking strategies are discussed later in this book.

Remember that answers to questions come from the passage. Remember that the Verbal Reasoning test does not ask you questions from your knowledge base. Answers will be either directly or

Table 2-2. Strategies for Reading the Passages

Read actively
Make a mental map
Identify topic sentences
Mark text
Answers come from passages
Check citations

indirectly stated. Because you may have previewed the question stems, you may be able to find the answers to questions as you read.

Check the citation at the end of the reading passage. Many Verbal Reasoning passages are drawn from books, journals, and other published works. If a passage is taken from a previously published piece, there will be a citation of the author, title, and date published. This citation gives you the title that the author assigned to the work, which frequently helps identify the answers to main idea questions.

Answering the Questions

There are several strategies for answering MCAT Verbal Reasoning questions (Table 2-3). This section provides question-answering techniques and identifies common traps to avoid.

Identifying Question Categories

As discussed in Chapter 1, there are six categories of Verbal Reasoning questions (Table 2-4). Assigning a category to each question can help you determine the correct answer.

Fact

Fact questions require you to report information that was specifically stated in the passage. Usually, the information is reworded or paraphrased in the answer choices. It is helpful to **go back to the passage** to find the information being discussed. If you made a mental map as you read or strategic notes in the margins of the paragraphs, it will be easy to find the answers to these questions.

The following phrases often appear in the stem of a fact question:

According to the passage . . .

Table 2-3. Strategies for Answering the Questions

Identify question category
Use process of elimination
Look for distractors
Identify qualifying words
Understand anatomy of choices
Transfer answers in blocks
Answer all questions

Table 2-4. Question Categories

1. Fact
2. Inference
3. Main idea
4. Tone
5. Application
6. Structure

The author states, says, asserts, claims, or declares...
The passage states, says, asserts, claims, or declares...
According to the author...

Traps to avoid when answering a fact question include:

- **Reading your own ideas into the passage or into the question or answer.** Remember to stay with the facts presented.
- **Looking for a complicated answer.** Generally, fact questions are straightforward and relatively simple. Do not make your task more difficult by "reading into" possible choices and confusing yourself.
- **Choosing answers that appear to be taken word-for-word from the passage**

Inference

These questions require that you understand what the passage implies rather than what it states specifically. Look for questions that ask you to make **assumptions** and **draw conclusions** on the basis of facts stated in the passage. To answer an inference question correctly, you first must know the basic facts of the passage, then organize appropriate facts into principles, and draw a conclusion from these principles that matches one of the answer choices.

Any question that requires you to give a reason for some statement or belief of the author is an inference question. The following phrases often appear in the stem of an inference question:

The passage suggests or implies...
It is the author's opinion or view...
One can assume...
It is the purpose of...
One can conclude...
It can be deduced or reasonably inferred...
The author most likely believes...

Traps to avoid when answering inference questions include:

- **Assuming that the answer can be found directly in the text.** Although all of the necessary information to answer a question correctly is within the text, you must go one step beyond the facts and draw a conclusion **based** on the facts.
- **Inserting your own opinions.** Although you must infer what the passage implies, you must do so on the basis of the materials given in the passage. Eliminate personal biases, and focus on ideas and information in the passage.

Main idea

This type of question asks you to **determine the central thesis** or **key concept** of the passage. To answer these questions correctly, you must **know the facts** of the passage, **organize those facts** into the basic principles of the text, **draw appropriate conclusions** regarding the relationship between the principles, and **determine the central thought** of the passage based on the relative importance of the principles contained in the passage.

The following phrases often appear in the stem of main idea questions:

The passage is primarily concerned with...
The central idea...
If you were to sum up the passage...

The main thought . . .
. . . best describes the passage . . .
The primary point . . .

Traps to avoid when answering main idea questions include:

- **Failing to include certain key facts in your decision-making process.** One of the best ways to keep all of the facts of a passage in mind before attempting to answer a main idea question is to write in the margin next to each paragraph one or two key words that summarize the thought contained in that paragraph. Then, consider the words you wrote, and think about a theme to link those words. Select the answer that most closely describes the theme supported by the key words.
- **Thinking that main idea questions are easy because, in a way, you are being asked to give a title to the passage.** These questions are often difficult, but if you avoid flowery or stylistic answers and stay with the main concepts contained in the passage, you should (with practice) be able to select the correct answer. Also, remember to look for a citation at the end of the passage. Frequently, looking at the citation title helps you arrive at the main idea.

Tone

Tone questions ask you to describe or identify the author's attitude in the passage. These questions usually refer to the tone of the whole passage. Answer these questions by thinking about the **feel** of the passage. Is it positive, negative, or neutral? How does the author seem to feel about the topic? Your first impression of the author's attitude is most likely the correct passage tone.

A **trap to avoid** when answering a tone question is:

- **Using your bias for the topic being discussed rather than the author's attitude.** It is critical that you think only about the author's opinion or feel for the topic.

Application

These questions ask you to take a concept or idea from the passage and apply it to a different situation. The key to answering these questions correctly is to **understand the concept** being described and **apply it, without significant change, to the new situation.** Try thinking of an analogy or a simple example of the concept to help you apply it to the new situation.

A **trap to avoid** when working with an application question is:

- **Taking a concept or idea that is presented in the passage and modifying it so that it does not "cleanly" apply to the new situation**

Structure

Structure questions ask you to describe the meaning or significance of a particular portion of the passage. The best way to answer these questions is to think of your **mental map** of the passage. Your mental map and any notations that you have made in the passage margins give you clues as to where to find information.

One **trap to avoid** when answering a structure question is:

- **Not making a mental map.** If you do not make a mental map of the passage as you read, you frequently will forget where ideas are stressed or mentioned. It is time-consuming to randomly search the passage for answers. When you waste time on the MCAT, you probably will not finish the test.

Process of Elimination

Use the process of elimination to find the best answer. Remember that an answer choice can be true and still be the wrong answer to a particular question. Your job is to find the **best** answer to each question.

Multiple Choice Questions

There will be four choices following each question (A–D). **Always use the process of elimination to answer each question.** For example, if you eliminate one of the four choices, your chance of answering a question correctly based on educated guessing goes from 25% to 33%. If you eliminate two choices, your chance of answering the question based on educated guessing alone goes all the way up to 50%. Although several answer choices may be correct statements, only one of the choices is the **best** correct statement. Always evaluate each choice to find which is best. If you are impulsive and do not evaluate each answer choice, you will often make an error and choose a correct statement that is not the best statement!

Extended Multiple Choice Questions

In this format, recall that the question is usually followed by three statements—I, II, and III. You choose which of those statements is correct and then choose the right answer. **Evaluate each statement based on its own merit.** If one of the statements is false or does not appropriately answer the question, eliminate it. When you eliminate the statement, eliminate the answer choices that contain that statement. This way, you are using the statements to strategically eliminate possible answer choices. Remember that for each answer choice you eliminate, your odds of getting any one question correct improve dramatically.

Distractors

Distractors are words or phrases in answer choices that are meant to distract you from the correct answer. **Look for distractors to help eliminate answer choices.** The test writers use distractors to design incorrect choices. Study the common distractors listed below. Always keep your eye out for distractors because they provide a way of eliminating incorrect choices!

Common Distractors

- **Choices that are outside the scope of the passage.** For example, if a choice to a question has little to do with the question or passage or appears to cover a peripheral topic, eliminate it. Also, eliminate any answer choice that goes too far beyond the coverage of the passage.
- **Choices that are too strong or too weak.** Some choices go too far and overstate a point from the passage. Other choices are too weak and do not make a key point sufficiently. Eliminate these types of choices.
- **Choices that are too broad or overgeneralized.** The test writers frequently test your ability to identify overstatements and improper assertions. If an answer choice makes too large a statement or is not specific enough, it is a distractor and should be eliminated.
- **Choices that make absolute statements.** Beware of choices that make emphatic statements. These options frequently are incorrect because a single exception is all that is needed to contradict the absolute statement. Remember that many of the passages on the MCAT cover nonscience areas and focus on discussion and inference. In these passage types, there is often an exception to almost any statement that can be made from the passage. In social science and humanities passages, rarely is there an instance in which an absolute statement is always true!
- **Choices that copy language from the passage with distorted meaning.** A common trick of test writers is to use manipulated wording from the passage to encourage the test taker to choose

an incorrect answer. Direct wording from a passage is rarely a correct answer choice. Test writers often modify a correct statement or idea from the passage and make it ambiguous or incorrect. This modified passage wording is then used as an answer choice. Always be suspicious of answer choices that appear to have phrases repeated from the passage. Evaluate the choices carefully to see if the context or meaning of the phrases from the passage has been changed.

- **Choices that appear "sexy."** Distractors often appear attractive and seductive. The choice may make a true statement, yet it might not directly answer the question. The majority of MCAT students who fall for these incorrect answer choices are the impulsive students. Never be impulsive! Remember that no matter how good an answer choice sounds, only the best answer is correct. **Do not fall for phrasing that sounds good but does not really answer the question.**

Always look for answer choices that contain distractors. Remember that distractors are placed by the test writers to lead you astray. A good way to eliminate answer choices is to take each choice and try to objectify it. Think if the choice makes a statement that is irrelevant to the passage or too generalized. Also, ask yourself if the choice makes a statement that is too strong or whether its tone conflicts with the tone of the passage.

Other Strategies

Look for questions containing qualifying words. Qualifying words give you clues to the correct answer. Examples of qualifying words include **best, most likely,** and **least.** Qualifying words are discussed in detail later in this book.

Understand the anatomy of answer choices. The test writers frequently invent choices that have little to do with the passage. These answer choices are not contradicted by anything in the passage, yet they are not supported either. **Always look for choices that do not appear to be supported.** Eliminate these. Also, eliminate answer choices that are contradicted. Keep in mind that the test writers rarely word correct choices with wording from the passage. Instead, **correct answer choices frequently are reworded to paraphrase the passage.** The purpose of this is to see if you can process the meaning of the choices.

Transfer your answers to the answer sheet in blocks. As you finish answering the questions to a passage, transfer all the answers from that passage to the answer sheet. This saves you at least 2–3 minutes over the course of the Verbal Reasoning test. In addition, this method decreases the risk that you will misnumber your answers.

Never leave questions unanswered. Remember that your score on Verbal Reasoning is based entirely on how many questions you answer correctly. There is no penalty for guessing. However, you should never need to randomly guess! If you reach a question that is difficult and you have no idea of the answer, try to eliminate one or more choices. If you can correctly eliminate even one choice, your educated guess has a 33% chance of being correct. Two correct eliminations raise the odds to 50%. This sure beats leaving the question unanswered and having a 0% chance of getting the question correct!

Now, let's move on to the next chapter. In chapter 3, you will figure out your reading speed and identify common problems you may have with your reading. Remember to review this chapter several times as you work through the Powerbuilder. It is critical to keep strategies in mind at all times!

Chapter 3

Reading Speed and Habits

The purpose of this chapter is to test your reading speed and comprehension ability. Also, some common reading habits that detract from speed and comprehension are discussed.

At this point, you need to test your reading speed and comprehension to determine your reading level. You will need a watch with a second hand and a pencil to mark down your reading times and answer comprehension questions. When you have read the passage and answered the questions, be sure to record your reading speed on the Goal Sheet (see page 221). This sheet allows you to measure your progress as you complete the chapters in this book.

Testing Speed and Comprehension

How to Compute Reading Rates

In addition to the record of your reading speed, keep track of your reading rate on other materials—your chemistry textbook, an article from the newspaper, a novel. You will become more aware of your reading rate and learn how your rate varies depending on what material you are reading. Use a small notebook to keep track of these rates.

To find out your reading rate, first determine the number of words on a page; then figure out the number of words you read per minute—this number equals your reading rate.

To figure the number of words on a page:

1. Choose any full page in a book. A full page has print from the top margin to the bottom margin, with no pictures.
2. On this page, choose three full lines (lines that begin at the left margin and end at the right margin).
3. Count all the words in these lines, including small words such as "I" and "the."
4. Divide the total number of words in these lines by three to get the average number of words in one line.
5. Count all the lines on the full page. Include every line, even if it contains only one word.
6. Multiply the total number of lines on the page (step 5) by the average number of words in a line (step 4) to get the approximate number of words on a page in that book.

MCAT Sample Passages: Test Your Ability

The first passage in this chapter is an example of one of the **easy passages** you could find in an MCAT Verbal Reasoning section. It is a passage drawn from a recent historical event. In the middle of this chapter you will read a passage of **medium difficulty.** At the end of the chapter, you will read a **difficult passage.** After completing this chapter, you will have a record of your initial reading speed on the different types of MCAT passages.

In addition, a short discussion of the content and form of each passage follows the answers to that passage's reading comprehension questions. This discussion is designed to get you used to thinking about the writing methods used for different passages.

Directions:
Record the times that you start and finish reading this passage in minutes and seconds. Subtract your starting time from your finishing time to find your total. Give yourself no more than 9 minutes to read the passage and answer the questions.

MCAT Practice Passage I

	Minutes	Seconds	
Your finishing time:			
Your starting time:			(subtract)
Your total time:			

Record your starting time now, and begin reading.

MCAT Practice Passage I (Easy)

Three of the most noted names in space exploration are Neil Armstrong, Michael Collins, and Edwin Aldrin. These astronauts left Earth in Apollo 11 on July 16, 1969. Their journey was one of the most amazing space expeditions ever. As they accelerated toward the moon, the world held its breath in anticipation. What used to be thought of as science fiction or fantasy, these brave men were about to attempt.

Four days after takeoff from Kennedy Space Center, Apollo 11 completed its trek and began to orbit the moon. Leaving Collins behind to man the mothership, Armstrong and Aldrin boarded the smaller space craft, named Eagle, and jettisoned toward the lunar surface. Everyone knew the dangers of the voyage, but no one could have predicted all the things that would go wrong.

As the Eagle's computers began their programmed descent, Armstrong and Aldrin looked for the landmarks they had memorized before leaving Earth. To their alarm, they realized most of these landmarks were behind them, and they were headed toward a deep crater lined with huge boulders. To add to their stress, communications with Earth were intermittently failing, and the Eagle's computer was warning of an overload. Armstrong calmly took control of the Eagle and guided it safely over two craters and numerous boulders before allowing the ship to resume its descent. In doing so, however, extra fuel was consumed, and a warning light came on at Mission Control. The ominous light meant that only 5% of the descent fuel remained. If the Eagle could not land within the next 94 seconds, the mission would have to be aborted.

As the seconds ticked by, Armstrong continued to negotiate the terrain, while Aldrin tensely reported instrument readings. Finally, with less than 20 seconds remaining and only about 2% of the descent fuel left, the Eagle made contact. The crew of the Apollo 11 felt both a sense of overwhelming joy and relief. At 4:17:43 eastern daylight-saving time, Mission Control received Armstrong's message, "Tranquillity Base here. The Eagle has landed."

While an estimated 25% of the world's population watched the lunar landing on television or listened to the event on the radio, Armstrong emerged from the hatch of the Eagle. He slowly climbed down the ladder, and as he gingerly set foot on the moon, he uttered the now-famous sentence, "That's one small step for man, one giant leap for mankind."

The trek of Apollo 11 was also a scientific one, and after a short period of relaxation and frolicking, the astronauts got to work. They collected soil samples and moon rocks, made observations, and set up a seismometer to measure moonquakes and a mirror to reflect back laser beams transmitted from Earth. They also unfurled a piece of aluminum foil to try to catch solar particles. We are normally protected from the solar wind, an ionized gas stream constantly emanating from the sun, by the Earth's magnetic field. The only time it reaches the Earth is when some leaks into the atmosphere near the polar regions, resulting in the luminescent auroras. The moon, however, does not have a strong magnetic field and is constantly bombarded by these atomic particles.

When Armstrong and Aldrin completed their experiments, they reentered the Eagle and returned to rendezvous with the mothership, Columbia. The three men then started their journey back to Earth. At home, the world was jubilant. We, the human race, had landed on the moon. These men had completed a journey that few people would have imagined possible 20 years before. In their voyage to the place that has fascinated generations of lovers and dreamers alike, these three men made history and brought hope to the world. No problem seemed quite as desperate or insurmountable because we had just successfully conquered the heavens and landed on the moon.

Word Count: 616 (See "How to Compute Reading Rates" in this chapter.)

Directions:
Record the time you have finished reading in the space provided at the beginning of this passage. Subtract your starting time from your finishing time to find out how long it took you to read it. This is your reading time.

Your reading time for MCAT Passage I is: ______________________________

Comprehension Questions

Answer the following comprehension questions for this passage. You may refer back to the passage as necessary.

1. It can be inferred from the passage that:

A. solar winds account for the differences between earthquakes and moonquakes.
B. Collins relayed messages between Mission Control and the Eagle when communications between the two broke down.
C. the Eagle might have crashed if Armstrong had not taken control of the descent from the Eagle's computers.
D. the rocks Armstrong and Aldrin brought back on the Eagle were the size of boulders.

2. Based on the information in the passage, one can conclude that:

A. the Eagle landed on the moon on July 20, 1969.
B. 25% of the world's population watched the live coverage of Neil Armstrong walking on the moon.
C. the huge boulders Armstrong and Aldrin saw when beginning their descent were obstacles they had overlooked when memorizing the moon's landmarks.
D. when the Eagle's computer warned of an overload, it was warning of low fuel.

3. Which of the following statements is supported by information in the passage?

I. The Earth's magnetic field is weaker at the polar regions.
II. The ascent of the Eagle required less fuel than the descent.
III. Armstrong and Aldrin conducted experiments in the Eagle before emerging from the hatch.

A. I only
B. I and II only
C. I and III only
D. I, II, and III

4. All of the following scenarios support the author's optimism at the end of the passage EXCEPT:

A. the European Economic Community reached new agreements regarding grain tariffs in December 1969.
B. Cold War tensions between the Soviet Union and the United States escalated after Apollo's voyage.
C. China opened its borders for the first visit ever of an American head of state shortly after Apollo's voyage.
D. Nixon's popularity soared at home and abroad after Apollo 11 returned.

5. The passage suggests that:

A. Tranquillity Base refers to Apollo 11.
B. the Earth has a greater magnetic field than the sun.
C. science was not very advanced 20 years ago.
D. Apollo 11 consisted of the Eagle and Columbia.

6. The best title for this passage might be:

A. "Three Men and a Moon."
B. "Americans Win the Race to Land on the Moon."
C. "The Incredible Voyage of Apollo 11."
D. "Who's that Man on the Moon?"

Directions:
Correct your answers by looking at the Answers and Explanations section. Allow 16.7 percentage points for each correct answer.

MCAT Practice Passage I Comprehension Score and Reading Time

Your comprehension test score ________%. Your reading time______________.

Your scores for MCAT Practice Passage I will serve as an **initial reference point** for the work you are going to do to improve your reading speed. It is important to keep track of how fast you read passages to see your progress. After each reading and comprehension test in this book, write down your rate and your comprehension score. Keep track of these rates on the Goal Sheet (see page 221), so you can compare scores as you progress.

Calculating Your Reading Speed on Practice Passage I

To figure your number of words per minute:

1. Count the number of pages you read. If you ended somewhere other than the bottom of a page, approximate how much of the page you read, one half, one third, and so on.
2. Multiply the number of pages you read by the number of words on a page to get the number of words you read. Because you read all these words in one minute, that figure is your rate, or words per minute.

For example, if the passage has 560 words on each page and you covered half of the page in a minute, your reading rate would be 280 words per minute:

560 (words) x ½ (pages) = 280 words per minute

MCAT Practice Passage I Reading Rate: ____________

While you are working through this book, make sure you calculate your reading rate every time you read a practice passage. Also, occasionally take your reading rate when you are reading outside material, and keep track of these rates in a notebook.

Discussion of MCAT Practice Passage I

NOTE: Discussion will follow Verbal Reasoning passages to get you thinking about the type of passage you are reading and the passage structure.

MCAT Passage I is a narrative passage. Narrative passages are usually among the easiest types of passages on the MCAT because they tend to be the most straightforward. The questions that follow the passages usually are fact, main idea, or structure questions. Narrative passages provide a record of events and activities that happen in a given period of time; these passages usually tell a story. The story of Apollo 11 and lunar landing is told here.

The first paragraph identifies the significance of the journey and the bravery of the astronauts involved. Note the use of these adjectives: *amazing, anticipation, brave.* The second paragraph identifies which astronauts boarded the Eagle and indicates that difficulties were to be encountered. The third paragraph outlines the difficulties, including boulders and a critical fuel shortage. Paragraph four provides resolution of the problems, and gives the reader a sense that lunar landing was barely achieved. The next paragraph briefly outlines Armstrong's first words on touching the moon's surface. Paragraph six describes experiments that Armstrong and Aldrin conducted. The terms *auroras* and *magnetic fields* are discussed in this paragraph. In the final paragraph, the significance of the Apollo 11 mission is emphasized.

Answers and Explanations to MCAT Practice Passage I

1. **C** Answer this question by evaluating each choice using the process of elimination. The question stem asks you to infer from the passage. This means that the correct answer choice will not be directly stated, but it will be implied. The third paragraph mentions that the Eagle was headed toward a crater and boulders. This was obviously a location where the crew did not want to land. Thus, Armstrong took control of the descent. It is logical that the Eagle might have crashed if Armstrong had not taken control of the spacecraft. Choices A, B, and D are not discussed or implied by the passage.

2. **A** Apollo 11 left Earth July 16 and then 4 days later, after starting to orbit the moon, the Eagle departed and landed on the moon. Choice B is incorrect because the passage stated that an estimated 25% of the world's population watched the moon walk on television **or** listened to coverage of the moon walk on radio. Choice C is not supported by the passage. The passage does not suggest or imply that the boulders were overlooked when memorizing the moon's landmarks; the passage does indicate that the landmarks that were memorized were behind them during descent. Choice D is incorrect because the third paragraph does not describe what the computer overload indicated.
3. **A** Statement I is correct. Paragraph six discusses the Earth's magnetic fields and the auroras produced by the solar winds as they leak through in the polar regions. The passage provides no evidence to support statement II. Although Armstrong and Aldrin conducted scientific experiments when they were on the moon's surface, there is no discussion of what they did in the Eagle before emerging. Thus, choice III is incorrect. By default, choice A is the best choice (I only).
4. **B** Note that this question stem asks for an exception to optimism. This means that the answer to this question should have a negative "charge." Choices A, C, and D indicate positive or optimistic situations, whereas choice B is a negative outcome or deteriorating situation.
5. **D** Answer this question by carefully evaluating each choice and eliminating incorrect or unsupported choices. Choice A is an attractive choice because Armstrong used the term *Tranquillity Base* when telling Mission Control that the Eagle had landed on the moon's surface. However, the use of Tranquillity Base is ambiguous. Was Armstrong describing the Eagle, Apollo 11, the moon, or himself? Do not eliminate choice A right away, but look for a better, clearer choice. Choice B can be eliminated because it is not supported by the passage. Choice C is a subjective statement that is arguable. Obviously, to send a mission to the moon, science must be fairly advanced. Choice D is clearly a true statement. Apollo 11 is the spaceship that left the Earth. The Eagle left the "mothership" and then rejoined the Columbia (the mothership). Choice D is clearly a true statement, whereas choice A is ambiguous. Thus, choice D is the best answer.
6. **C** When asked about the best title for a passage, the best choice is the one that summarizes the passage and captures the author's tone. Choices A and D are almost comical. They do not capture the true gist and attitude of the passage. Choice B does not accurately summarize the passage because space program competition was not discussed in this passage. Choice C is the best choice by default. As a general rule, the most likely answers to best title-type questions are those that avoid stylistic or verbose titles.

Common Reading Habits

Identifying Common Reading Habits, Blocks, and Attitudes

Everyone has different reading habits. If you become more aware of your own habits as a reader, it is easier to figure out what might be slowing you down. Readers can be classified into three different groups: **motor, auditory,** and **sight readers.** Most people are a combination of all three. Although these habits will not always detract from your reading, it is good to recognize them.

Motor Readers

Motor readers move some part of their body as they read. Reading and body movement are synchronized into one process. If you take away the movement—chewing gum, twirling hair, jiggling legs or feet—the reading style is disrupted. Generally, **body movement slows down reading speed.**

You may not be aware that you are moving as you read. Have someone watch you read for five minutes to determine if you are a motor reader. If you are, be aware of the movement as you read, and stop yourself from doing it! This takes discipline and practice, but it may result in a faster reading speed.

Auditory Readers

Auditory readers rely on hearing the words. Even when auditory readers are silently reading, they form the words with their lips as if they were speaking them. This slows down reading because the reading is allowed to happen only as fast as the reader can speak. This type of auditory vocalization occurs at several different levels. Some readers actually **say the words aloud** as they read, but they are unaware they are doing this. When questioned about this tendency, the readers may explain that they have to say the words, or else they will not understand what they are reading. Other readers **say words under their breath** as they read. This slows down reading because the reader can only digest words as they are mumbled.

Some readers do not actually say or mumble words as they read them. These readers actually **hear each word mentally** as they read. Hearing every single word works well when reading poetry or a love letter—when you want to savor the sound of language. However, when you are reading for information—such as on the MCAT—you want to be able to digest and comprehend as much text as quickly as possible.

Sight Readers

Sight readers instantly understand the printed symbol without auditory association. This is the **fastest form** of reading because it does not rely on sound or physical movement. Sight readers see a word or a group of words and instantly perceive a visual image with the meaning associated with the printed symbol. If you are a sight reader, you will probably be able to read much faster than motor or auditory readers.

Take time to think about your habits as a reader. When you are aware of these habits, you will be able to focus on ways to change them.

Other Reading Habits

Some readers tend to **overanalyze** what they are reading. However, not all the material in a passage is worth analyzing. Some parts of a passage are more important than others. You can choose when to analyze closely and when to skim over material to get a general idea of the information.

Other readers read **word for word** instead of for ideas. The human brain can process 800 words a minute. So why do most of us read at a much slower rate than this? Because we read word for word. This type of reading causes our minds to wander.

People also read without total concentration. They allow themselves to become **distracted.** It is up to you to decide that when you sit down to read, you are going to give reading material your total attention. Be aware of your own stamina, and take a short break when your attention wanders. Try reading in half-hour intervals at first, taking 5-minute breaks to rest your eyes and walk around. This may seem time-consuming, but taking breaks actually improves your reading efficiency because you will be refreshed and have a clear head during the time you spend reading. As you practice more, your ability to concentrate over longer periods will increase. It will not take you long to work up to the 85-minute testing period of the Verbal Reasoning test.

Maybe you recognize some of your own reading habits and tendencies in those just described. Make a note of your habits in the space provided below, and try to avoid them. Realize that these habits are slowing you down and may affect your test score.

Now, get out your pencil and your watch again, and give your full attention to the second MCAT passage in this chapter. This is a **medium difficulty passage**—quite a bit more difficult than the first passage. What makes this passage difficult is the amount of **inference** you will have to make in answering the questions. Read very carefully. Mark your beginning and ending times; then answer the comprehension questions. Try to use the basic strategies that were presented in Chapter 2. Remember, **be an active reader. Concentrate!**

Directions:
Record the times that you start and finish reading this passage in minutes and seconds. Subtract your starting time from your finishing time to find your total time.

MCAT Practice Passage II

	Minutes	Seconds	
Your finishing time:			
Your starting time:			(subtract)
Your total time:			

Record starting time now, and begin reading.

Try to finish reading this passage in 3–4 minutes. Allow another 5 minutes to answer the questions.

MCAT Practice Passage II (Medium Difficulty)

In his introduction to *The Classic Slave Narratives,* Henry Louis Gates, Jr., claims that "in literacy lay true freedom for the slave." Clearly, literacy was viewed as an empowering tool by both blacks and whites in the pre-Civil War South, as white slave owners made literacy illegal for their black slaves. While slavery remained legal, it was illegal for anyone to teach a slave how to read and write. One particular man, Frederick Douglass, best epitomizes the irony that literacy and empowerment brought the slave.

In Frederick Douglass' slave narrative, collected in the Gates anthology, Douglass tells how he was able to become literate despite the laws against it and how literacy aided him in his quest for freedom. One of Douglass' white mistresses, a first-time slave owner, taught Douglass the alphabet. Douglass pursued this learning with interest but not with real enthusiasm until his lessons were ended abruptly. When Douglass' master realized that his wife was teaching their slave to read and write, he instantly forbade her to continue in the endeavor. Scolding her, Douglass' master explained that literacy would ruin a slave–it would "unfit" him or her to be a slave. Upon overhearing this reprimand, Douglass realized that power lay in literacy, and he began to seek other means to continue his education.

Douglass was a bright, compulsive, and driven man. Exchanging bread for elementary lessons, Douglass coaxed poor white children in lower socioeconomic-class neighborhoods to teach him how to read and write. When they called him "lucky" for having plenty to eat, he told them they were the truly lucky ones—they were freeing their minds in school, and they would grow up physically free as well. At age 18 years, the white children, even the poor, would become their own masters. Eventually, Douglass became fully literate, and he began to teach other slaves to read and write whenever possible.

In his narrative, Douglass describes becoming literate as an awakening. For the first time, Douglass became aware of a universe outside the world of slavery. He also realized the full extent of the injustices of slavery. He began to understand that his personhood had been stolen, and he began to want that personhood back.

In the course of his readings, Douglass learned the meaning of a word he had heard but had never understood; that word was *abolition*. Douglass learned that there were white people in North America who decried slavery. He realized that there was a place to which he could escape, and there were people in the North who might help him. Although clearly empowering in many ways, literacy was also debilitating for Douglass. Unable to escape until several years after he became literate, Douglass was forced to endure mental and spiritual tribulations because of his newly acquired knowledge. In many ways, his awakening made his condition as a slave even more miserable than when he remained ignorant. Douglass had to endure the realization of his potential freedom without being able to attain it.

Adapted from James MacFearson, *The Narratives of Frederick Douglass.* © 1995 by Prentice-Hall, Inc.

Word count: 490

Directions:
Record the time you finished reading in the space provided at the beginning of the passage. Subtract your starting time from your finishing time to find out how long it took to read the passage. Then, figure your reading rate.

Your reading rate is: ______________________________

Comprehension Questions

1. According to Gates, the term *true freedom* as used in the passage is:

A. strength.
B. escape from physical bondage.
C. awakening.
D. knowledge.

2. Douglass continues to seek an education after he hears his master forbid it because Douglass is:

A. shrewd.
B. disobedient.
C. rebellious.
D. tricky.

3. The passage as a whole implies that literacy "unfits" a slave because it makes the slave:

A. miserable.
B. angry.
C. intelligent.
D. realize his or her personhood.

4. It might be said that literacy not only "frees the mind" but also:

A. connects people.
B. breaks the body.
C. destroys the spirit.
D. embitters masters.

5. Based on the passage, mental freedom without physical freedom is:

A. true freedom.
B. slavery.
C. tortuous.
D. literacy.

6. The passage as a whole implies that ignorance is:

A. bliss.
B. peace of mind.
C. painful.
D. debilitating.

7. According to Douglass, freedom means:

A. literacy.
B. peace of mind.
C. physical freedom.
D. knowledge and control.

Directions:
Correct your answers by looking at the Answers and Explanations section. Allow 14.6 percentage points for each correct answer.

MCAT Practice Passage II Comprehension Score and Reading Rate

Your comprehension test score ________%. *Your reading rate* ____________.

Discussion of MCAT Practice Passage II

This passage is an **expository passage;** it explains how Douglass was able to become literate despite the laws against it. As in all expository passages, this passage provides information about a subject. Also, notice that this passage has a citation. The citation shows that a third-party author recently wrote the article or book from which this passage was drawn. The generic name of the piece given in the citation, *The Narratives of Frederick Douglass,* also indicates that the passage provides information on the writings of Douglass, rather than arguments or opinions of the author.

Each paragraph in this expository passage has a different purpose. The first paragraph describes the importance of literacy in the pre-Civil War South and indicates that it was illegal to teach slaves how to read. Paragraph two provides the background behind Douglass' earliest reading lessons and discusses Douglass' realization that literacy equals power. Paragraph three outlines Douglass' interaction with poor, white children and his exchanging bread with them for reading lessons. Paragraph four emphasizes Douglass' awakening on the injustices of slavery. The final paragraph discusses Douglass' thoughts, tribulations, and the abolition of slavery.

Answers and Explanations to MCAT Practice Passage II

1. **D** To answer this question, look for the place in the passage where the work of Gates is discussed. A quotation of Gates in the first paragraph indicates that "true freedom" is acquired through literacy. Literacy is linked implicitly to knowledge in paragraph four. This makes choice D supported by the passage. Choices A and B sound good at first glance, but they are not supported directly in the passage. Choice C is an attractive choice because the term *awakening* is discussed in paragraphs four and five. Impulsive students tend to be drawn to choice C. However, this choice should be eliminated because the discussion of awakening is not linked to Gates.
2. **A** Ask yourself how the author portrays Douglass. Look carefully at paragraph two. Notice that Douglass does not disobey his master just for the sake of rebellion. He disobeys his master because he realizes that there must be power in literacy. Based on the tone of the passage, one should expect that the author would describe Douglass in a positive light for this behavior. Note that choice A, shrewd, is the least negative of the choices. By shrewd, we should believe that the author means sharp, keen, or astute. Disobedience, rebellious, and tricky are definitely negative in connotation and should be eliminated as choices.
3. **D** The passage leads one to believe that Douglass feels slavery is unjust. Paragraph four emphasizes the awakening and the realization of Douglass that his personhood had been stolen. What is it that "unfits" a slave? Education and literacy give the slave power to understand that his or her personhood has been stolen.
4. **A** This is an inference question. To answer this question, determine what literacy brought to Douglass. In paragraph five, note that literacy opened up a network of abolitionists for Douglass. This clearly

connected Douglass to new people in the North. This supports choice A. Choices B, C, and D all carry negative connotations. The second half of paragraph five describes ways in which literacy debilitated Douglass. However, none of these choices (B, C, D) are described in this paragraph.

5. **C** Paragraph five states: "Unable to escape until several years after he became literate, Douglass was forced to endure mental and spiritual tribulations. . . ." This section of paragraph five suggests that remaining in slavery after his awakening is "miserable" for Douglass. Which word is closest to miserable? Choice C, or tortuous, is the best word here.

6. **D** This is another inference question. The answer to this question is implied throughout the passage. Literacy, and therefore knowledge, is empowering. Thus, ignorance must be disempowering, and "debilitating" is the closest answer offered. Choices A and B are incorrect based on the context of this passage. Ignorance carries a strong negative connotation in this passage. Although choice C carries a negative connotation, it is not the best choice because it is too vague and is not discussed in the passage.

7. **D** In the third paragraph, Douglass describes two freedoms: freedom of the mind and physical freedom. Based on the passage, literacy alone is not freedom, so eliminate choice A. Similarly, physical freedom alone is not complete freedom. Thus, eliminate choice C. Choice B is not discussed or supported in the passage. Choice D is best because literacy is but a means toward mental freedom (knowledge) and physical freedom (control) for Douglass.

Concentration

To improve your reading speed and comprehension, you need to know the purpose of your reading and why concentration is important. When reading something that interests us, reading goes quickly. Unfortunately, not all reading we do is about subjects that fascinate us. Some of the topics in the Verbal Reasoning passages may not be familiar or even interest you. However, you must continue reading with concentration in order to complete the test. Your purpose in reading these MCAT passages is to get through the test, answering as many questions correctly as possible. Keep this purpose in the forefront of your mind as you read. **Remember that the desire to succeed is a great tool for concentration!**

As you read a passage, think about what the author is trying to say. Formulate your own questions about the topic. For example, what is the main idea, tone, or contradiction of the passage? Think of the writer as a person trying to get a message across to you. What kinds of questions would you ask that person?

In the next chapter, we will practice this kind of concentration at greater length, and you will have the opportunity to practice your comprehension with a wide variety of texts.

The following passage is the most **difficult** practice passage in this chapter. Remember to concentrate.

Directions:
Record the times that you start and finish reading this passage in minutes and seconds. Subtract your starting time from your finishing time to find your total.

MCAT Practice Passage III

	Minutes	Seconds	
Your finishing time:			
Your starting time:			(subtract)
Your total time:			

Write starting time now, and begin reading.

Try to read the passage in 3–4 minutes. Allow 5 minutes to answer the questions.

MCAT Practice Passage III (Difficult)

What is wrong with the young people of today? Young people are uneasy. They do not recognize their right to be young. It is as though youth were not an age of life, but a class phenomenon, an unduly prolonged childhood, a spell of irresponsibility accorded to the children of the well-to-do. The workers go without transition from adolescence to manhood. And it really does look as though our age, which is in the process of eliminating the tightly knit upper classes, is also eliminating that abstract period of which people have always said, "It will have its fling." Most of my former students have married early because they felt ashamed of their youth and of the leisure that was once in fashion.

They have become fathers before they have finished their studies. They still receive money from their families at the end of each month, but it is not enough. They have to give lessons or perform odd jobs as part-time workers. In one way, they are like kept-women in a traditional foreign culture, and in another, like "home workers." They no longer take the time, as we did at their age, to play about with ideas before adopting one set in particular.

They are fathers and citizens, they vote, they must commit themselves. This is probably not a bad thing. It is fitting, after all, that they be asked to choose immediately for or against man, for or against the masses. But if they choose the first side, their difficulties begin, because they are persuaded that they must strip themselves of their subjectivity. If they consider doing this, it is for reasons which remain subjective, as they are still inside. They take counsel with themselves before plunging themselves into the water and, as a result, the more seriously they contemplate abandoning subjectivity, the greater the importance it assumes in their eyes.

However, that is not the end of it. They are now told to choose between materialism and idealism; they are told that there is nothing in-between and that it must be one or the other. Now, to most of them, the principles of materialism seem philosophically false; they are unable to understand how matter could give rise to the idea of matter. Nevertheless, they protest that they utterly reject idealism. They know that it acts as a myth for the propertied classes and that it is not a rigorous philosophy but a rather vague kind of thinking whose function is to mask reality or to absorb it into the idea. "It doesn't matter," they are told by their professors. "Since you are not materialists, you will be idealists in spite of yourselves, and if you rebel against this label given to you by your professors, you will find yourselves the victims of a more subtle and all the more dangerous illusion."

Thus, they are hounded even in their thoughts, which are poisoned at the source, and they are condemned to serve unwillingly a philosophy they dislike, or to adopt out of discipline a doctrine in which they are unable to believe. They have lost the carefree quality characteristic of their age without acquiring the certainty of maturity. They are no longer at their leisure and yet they cannot commit themselves. The most difficult thing for me to witness as their professor, is their conflict with the two opposing forces that most young people battle against in their struggle to determine their own destiny: materialism versus idealism.

Jean R. Bresbou, *Materialism and Idealism: The Controversy.*

Word Count: 518

Directions:
Record the time you have finished reading in the space provided at the beginning of this passage. Subtract your starting time from your finishing time to find out how long it took you to read it. This is your reading time.

Your reading time for MCAT Practice Passage III is: ______________________

Comprehension Questions

Answer the following comprehension questions for this passage. You may refer back to the passage as necessary.

1. According to the passage, the author favors the values of:

A. materialism.
B. idealism.
C. spiritualism.
D. rigorous philosophy.

2. Based on information presented in the passage, which principle(s) would young people most likely react to negatively?

I. Idealism
II. Marriage
III. Materialism

A. I only
B. I and II only
C. I and III only
D. I, II, and III

3. At the time this piece was written, the author believed that young people suffered from:

A. marriage at too advanced an age.
B. not enough responsibility.
C. an emphasis on materialism.
D. lost youth.

4. The passage suggests that young people have to select among several difficult choices. These choices do NOT include:

A. serving a philosophy that they dislike.
B. serving their own belief system.
C. serving a philosophy that they are unable to believe.
D. choosing for or against man, or for or against the masses.

5. If the author of this passage were to run for political office, one would expect him to run as a:

A. democrat or republican.
B. capitalist.
C. materialist.
D. socialist.

6. The choice of "man" as described in the passage is best linked to:

A. the coming of age.
B. the gain of materialism.
C. the loss of subjectivity.
D. the choice of idealism.

Directions:
Correct your answers by looking at the Answers and Explanations. Allow 16.7 percentage points for each correct answer.

MCAT Practice Passage III Comprehension Score and Reading Rate

Your comprehension test score ________%. *Your reading rate* ____________

(Note: Do not get upset! Expect that your reading time and comprehension may be a little lower on this difficult passage than on the easier passages.)

Discussion of MCAT Practice Passage III

This passage represents what a difficult, philosophical passage on the MCAT might look like. This is an argumentative passage. The author presents a position on a controversial topic. Some of the points of the author are explicitly stated, whereas others are implicitly stated. As with many philosophical passages that have appeared on the MCAT, this passage has some ambiguity and inference that you must work through. The best way to do this is to make a mental map of what ideas and discussion are presented in each paragraph of the passage. Also, make notes in the margins opposite each paragraph of the passage.

Without question, this passage contains both philosophy and political undertones. It carries a socialistic tone. Note the use of these key words: *workers, underclass, materialism, idealism,* and *propertied classes.* Also, note that the citation at the end of the passage gives a title that provides some clues as to the content of the passage. First, the citation points to a controversy between materialism and idealism. Make sure to look for a discussion of this controversy in the passage. Second, the copyright date of the citation gives you a clue that this is a passage that was adapted from the postwar period. This most likely explains the political nature of the piece.

Based on the content of the passage, the author appears to be a philosopher and professor who teaches in a university. The passage presents an argument in which the author discusses the difficult decision between materialism versus idealism that young people must ponder. He also discusses the challenges that young people of the period face. The first paragraph focuses on the concept of lost youth and gives the reader the suggestion that the society about which the author is writing is in the process of removing its upper classes. In the second paragraph, the author discusses how young people have taken on the responsibilities of adulthood, yet are still children in a way. They still are dependent on the older generation. In the last sentence of the second paragraph, he also states that young people do not take the time to ponder and mature. In the third paragraph, the author states that young people must choose between "man" and the "masses." If they choose man, we are told that they must strip themselves of their subjectivity. Perhaps the author is referring to man as a current leadership, whereas masses refers to the working class or popular alternative leadership. The author does appear to link man with a negative connotation, by linking it with the loss of subjectivity. In paragraph four, materialism versus idealism is introduced. The author presents the concept that most young people of the time find materialism philosophically false, yet they totally reject idealism for its ambiguity and "mask" on reality. However, in the final sentence of this paragraph, we are told that their professors label them as idealists by default. In the final paragraph, the author strongly points out that young people have a choice to either serve a philosophy they dislike and which is poisoned, or serve a philosophy that they are unable to believe. In the final sentence of the passage, the author indicates that he has had difficulty witnessing the struggle young people have had in choosing between materialism and idealism. He indicates that he has made his own choice, and we must infer from the passage that as a professor, he has chosen the idealistic route.

Answers and Explanations to MCAT Passage III

1. **B** Answer this question by inference. The author states that he is a professor in the final paragraph. In the last sentence of the fourth paragraph, the author suggests that professors label students as idealists. Thus, it makes sense that the author favors the values of idealism. Another clue is the choice of words and tone that the author uses to describe those with material goods and those without. It appears that the author's focus is less on material goods and more on ideals and values. Choice A is not supported by inference in this passage. Choice C is not discussed at all. Choice D can also be eliminated. Although the author may support rigorous philosophy, we have no direct evidence in the passage to support this.
2. **C** Statements I and III are supported in the passage. In the fourth paragraph, it is explained that young people react negatively to both materialism and idealism, although not to the same degree. The author states: "Now, to most of them, the principles of materialism seem philosophically false; they are unable to understand how matter could give rise to the idea of matter. Nevertheless, they protest that they utterly reject idealism." Statement II is not supported in the passage. At the end of the first paragraph, the author discusses that most of his young students have married early. The motivations for marriage, as discussed by the author, are not important here.
3. **D** It is important to answer this question without inserting your own opinions. Find the best answer by carefully considering the arguments presented in this passage. Evaluate each choice based on its own merit. Choice A is incorrect because the author believes that young people marry at too young an age. He also points out that young people carry too much responsibility without the time to ponder, mature, and live out their youth, thus making choice B incorrect. In the fourth paragraph, the author states that young people find materialism philosophically false, thus making choice C incorrect. In several places in the passage, the author alludes to the concept of "lost youth."
4. **B** In the final paragraph, the author strongly points out that young people have a choice to either serve a philosophy they dislike and which is poisoned, or serve a philosophy that they are unable to believe. This eliminates choices A and C. The third paragraph also indicates that young people must make another series of choices. The passage states that, "they be asked to choose immediately

for or against man, for or against the masses." Thus, choice D is incorrect. Although choice B appears at first glance to be a reasonable choice that young people should make, it is not stated in the passage anywhere. This is the best answer to this question by the process of elimination. Note that the other choices were eliminated quickly because they were all directly stated in the passage.

5. **D** This is also an inference question. The author voices his idealistic views and imparts an attitude supporting the working classes. Class commentary is used throughout the passage with the use of words selected to point out class distinction: *workers, underclass,* and *propertied classes.* This is most consistent with socialistic views.

6. **C** In this question, you are asked about the use of the term *man*. Carefully skim the passage to find the term used in the third paragraph. Note these two important sentences from the third paragraph: "It is fitting, after all, that they be asked to choose immediately for or against man, for or against the masses. But if they choose the first side, their difficulties begin, because they are persuaded that they must strip themselves of their subjectivity." The link between "man" and loss of subjectivity is clearly stated. Choices A, B, and C are not directly related to the use of the term *man* in this passage.

By now, you should have an idea of some areas you need to focus on; you might read passages quickly but lose accuracy in answering comprehension questions. Or, you might read passages more slowly, but get all the answers right in the comprehension section. Make it your goal to be fast and accurate in both reading passages and answering questions about them. This, of course, takes a lot of practice. So let's keep going! In the next chapter, we will focus on comprehension techniques for MCAT passages.

Chapter 4

Context and Meaning: Improving Comprehension of MCAT Passages

In this chapter, we will focus on the meaning of a passage as a whole, rather than the individual words that comprise a passage. The goal is to decrease your focus on individual words so that you can determine the main idea and context of the passage more quickly.

When you concentrate on individual, unimportant words in a passage, you significantly reduce your speed and concentration. You must try to **concentrate on the important (or key) words in the passage** because these words carry the meaning. In this chapter, you will learn the techniques to locate words that appear to carry important meaning and focus less on **"filler" words** (words that fill in gaps between important words).

You may wonder how the meaning of a passage can be understood without reading the filler words. **Your brain automatically fills in the meanings of words without actually reading them.** Try quickly reading this passage:

Cohabitation

Some social scientists believe living together equals x loss xx social institutions, xxx consequently, a xxxx of xxx structure xx society. Xxx idea xx x permanent commitment to xxxxxxx person has lost xxx meaning, some argue. Others argue xxxx cohabitation weakens xxx family xxx erodes xxx xxxxx of obligation xx love xxx working relationships.

A significant number of words have been left out, but you most likely were able to fill in the gaps by association, looking at the surrounding words for context. You can train yourself to do this with any text, without crossing out words. Specific techniques for key-word searching are covered in Chapter 5.

When you glanced at this passage, you probably read the title. Reading the title was useful because it gave you a **framework** or a **context** that limited your ideas about the meaning of the passage. Using that context, you were able to fill in the gaps in a passage about the topic of cohabitation. You were reading for the **main idea,** and this made you read more quickly.

However, most MCAT passages do not have titles, so extracting the main idea may be more difficult than just reading a title. There are three other ways to understand the main idea of a passage. Let's look at the three approaches that can help you form a context about the main idea of a passage.

Context and Main Idea: Three Important Strategies

There are three basic strategies that can help determine the context and main idea of a passage. These techniques include **skimming and titling the passage, acknowledging the source of the passage,** and **skimming the comprehension questions before reading the passage.**

Strategy 1: Skimming and Titling

As soon as your eyes read text, you automatically form ideas about the information the text contains. If the text has a byline, you make assumptions about the contents of the text based on what you know of the author. For example, if you see that an article is written by Andy Rooney, you can assume the piece will be humorous and probably political. MCAT passages generally do not have bylines, so you must look to the words to provide context. By initial skimming or just reading the topic sentences of a passage, you usually can determine the tone of the author and the subject of the passage.

Reading for the main idea, with the intent to put a title on the passage, can help you place the passage in context. When you skim through a passage, the first thing you should do is look for a possible thesis. Recall that a **thesis** is a sentence that sums up what the passage is about. **Often, the thesis will be found toward the end of the first paragraph.**

Drill: Strategy 1

Skim through this paragraph, and perform the following tasks:

1. Identify the thesis.
2. Give the paragraph a title.

Last year it happened again. The controversy came to the forefront. The people surrounded by or even remotely interested in college football stirred up the question of who is Number One in college football. It was argued: "Should the old way of voting with coaches and writers remain, or should a new playoff system take its place?" Despite arguments to the contrary, a playoff system should determine the national championship in college football.

Discussion of Strategy 1 Drill

1. In this paragraph, the last sentence is an argumentative statement, stating an opinion. This last sentence is the thesis on which the essay focuses. The thesis tells you as the reader what to expect in the passage, and identifying it increases the clarity of the passage.
2. A range of titles are possible. The key is to make sure that your title puts the passage in context. Based on the thesis, a possible title might be, "College Football Playoffs Are Necessary." This title summarizes the idea given in the thesis and, consequently, the argumentative idea of the passage. Make note of your title by penciling it in above the passage. This title will help you focus as you read more carefully and answer comprehension questions.

Strategy 2: Acknowledging the Source of the Passage

Always look for a citation! When you work on the Verbal Reasoning section of the MCAT, look to the end of each passage, just before the questions begin. Is there information that looks like this?

Adapted from John Allen Paulos, *Innumeracy: Mathematical Illiteracy and Its Consequences.* © 1988 by John Allen Paulos.

Yes! Most of the time, MCAT passages are adapted from copyrighted books, articles, and periodicals. We have noticed that **more than 75%** of the passages on the MCAT are followed by a citation of the author, title of the piece from which the work was taken, and copyright date. Actually, on the recently released set of real MCAT questions from Practice Test III (AAMC, 1995), all nine of the Verbal Reasoning passages were followed by citations! This is great news for you because citations provide you with a good deal of information.

The bibliographical information that directly follows MCAT passages automatically gives you important context for the passage because you can learn from which larger piece of work this passage was taken. Look for a citation before you begin reading.

What to Look for in a Citation

1. **Do you recognize the author's name?** Sometimes passages are taken from famous literary works. If you recognize the author and know something about the author's style, you have an advantage. If you do not recognize the author, move on to the next clue—the title.
2. **What is the title of the piece from which the passage was adapted?** The title of the source is the **most critical** piece of information given in the citation. Frequently, the title of the source gives you hints about the **main idea, attitude,** and **tone** of the passage. The title of the piece is often a one-sentence summary of the entire passage. If nothing else, spend a few seconds thinking about the title given in the citation.
3. **What is the source of the passage?** Is the source a book or a magazine? What do you know about the particular bias or political slant of the book or magazine? **Thinking about the source of the passage will put the passage into context.** Give the piece your own title as well, but only after you have acknowledged the original source.
4. **What is the copyright date?** Knowing when a passage was written gives you an **idea of the attitude at the time of publication.** For example, a passage discussing the role of women in society with a copyright date of 1950 will lead you to believe that the passage contains opinions and values that may be different now.

Citation Drill

Given below are some citations similar to those appearing on recent MCAT Verbal Reasoning tests. Just by studying the citations, try to determine the **main idea** of the passage and the probable **tone** or **attitude** of the author. See if you can determine whether or not the passage will be **expository, narrative,** or **argumentative.** A discussion of each citation and its corresponding passages will follow.

Citation 1: From G.M. Watson, American Government: *The Ever Changing Liberalism in Our Politics and Public Policy.* © 1990, US News and World Report.

Discussion of Citation 1

On first glance, the name of the author does not appear familiar. However, the title of the source of this passage tells you a lot about the likely content. First, notice that the author's title appears to be pointing out how our politics are becoming more liberal. It appears that this author is probably sensitive to liberalism and may be critical of it. The use of the term *ever changing* suggests that the author may have some concerns about the advancement of liberal politics. Also, notice the source of this passage. It was drawn from *US News and World Report,* a magazine that you may know generally supports conservative politics. The passage is likely argumentative, where the author presents and defends his position on the controversial topics of politics.

Citation 2: Adapted from Pablo Picasso, *Frivolity, Understanding, and the Demise of Serious Art Education.* © 1994, by the Pablo Picasso Art Educational Foundation.

Discussion of Citation 2

The author's name sure looks familiar! This author appears to be a family member of the great artist, Pablo Picasso. This belief is supported by the source of the piece, the Pablo Picasso Art Educational Foundation. The title of the piece provides a lot of information; it suggests that art education is or has been deteriorating. The word *frivolity* implies some sort of flightiness. Perhaps the author believes that there is a misunderstanding of the meaning of art. Obviously, the charge of this piece is negative and judgmental. The author may be defending the work of Pablo Picasso and some misunderstanding or lack of appreciation of his work. Note that the passage was drawn from recent writings. The passage is likely argumentative.

Citation 3: From James Johnson, *The Immortal Wilderness We Need.* © 1994 by James Johnson.

Discussion of Citation 3

The author's name is not familiar. The title of the piece suggests that the topic of the passage will be about the wilderness. There appears to be an opinion expressed in the title. The adjective *immortal* leads you to believe that the wilderness will, or should, live forever. The author wants us to believe that an eternal wilderness is necessary. Maybe the author is worried about our deteriorating wilderness lands; thus, the attitude of the piece may have an environmentalist tone. The passage probably is drawn from a book or independent work because no magazine or other credit is given. The passage likely tells a story (narrative) or provides information about a subject (expository/informative).

Citation 4: From A.R. Lopes, *The Burned Earth: How Heat from the Earth's Core Triggers Surface Upheaval.* © 1995 by the National Institute for Geologic Studies.

Discussion of Citation 4

The author's name is not familiar. This passage clearly is about the natural sciences (geology). The title of the piece tells you what this passage is all about. The main idea may be contained in the title, so if the questions ask you about the main idea of the passage, be sure to refer to this citation. The passage is recent and copyrighted by a national study group in geology. This means that the passage will likely contain detailed scientific facts and be expository/informative.

Citation 5: From T. Leary, *A Case for Legalization of Substances.* © 1970 by T. Leary.

Discussion of Citation 5

To some of you, this author may be familiar. The author of this passage was the late Timothy Leary. Dr. Leary was a Harvard professor who left a professorship at Harvard to advocate exploring the mind with drugs. He promoted substance use (e.g., LSD) and was a controversial figure in the late 1960s and early 1970s. The title of the piece suggests that the author will discuss the legalization of drug substances. Even if you did not recognize the author, it is fairly obvious that the passage will be argumentative in favor of substance legalization. The date that this piece was written also gives you important clues as to the political attitude of the time. In 1970, drug use in the United States was escalating, and there was much debate about drugs and war. Remember to think about the biases of a known author, and look at the wording of the citation title carefully.

Strategy 3: Skimming the Questions Before Reading the Passage

Reading through the question stems before you read the passage will help you look for **specific information** and **key words** as you read. For instance, if you see that several of the questions focus on a particular kind of "phenomenon," you need to look for the specific definition of the phenomenon within the passage, and pay special attention to any examples the passage uses as they pertain to the questions.

Also, the kinds of questions pertaining to a passage can tell you what kind of passage you will read. The three main types of passage in the MCAT verbal reasoning section are **narrative, expository,** and **argumentative** (see Chapter 1, Types of Writing). The kinds of questions you will be asked on each of these types of passage will help you to determine what to expect in the passage—again, you will be able to put the passage into some kind of context based on the kinds of questions asked.

Here are examples of questions asked about an **argumentative** passage. Look at the passage after you examine some of the questions. **Notice how the questions themselves can give a strong sense of the content of the reading.**

1. The author of the passage:

A. promotes Choice.
B. is undecided about Choice.
C. is indifferent about Choice.
D. rejects Choice.

Even though you cannot yet define "Choice," you can infer clearly from this question that the passage promotes a certain viewpoint, which indicates an argumentative passage.

2. The passage implies that which of the following is the real problem behind the current educational crisis?

A. Government policy
B. Economic disparity
C. Political rhetoric
D. Enrollment

Again, this question infers that a specific point of view is expressed in the passage, and you will be able to look specifically for that point of view in your reading.

3. According to the author of the passage, the Choice plan would widen the gap between the rich and the poor because:

A. vouchers would not be large enough.
B. private schools are all in the suburbs.
C. the poor live in the inner city.
D. public schools are all in the inner city.

This question is asking about one of the author's supports for the argument.

From these three questions, you can conclude that the passage that you are about to read is argumentative. You should expect the passage to try to convince or persuade you toward or away from a viewpoint. Always ask yourself, **what is the purpose of the passage?** This is yet another way to put the reading into context because you then know what kind of information you are supposed to get out of the reading.

The passage follows in full. Try the skimming and titling technique as you quickly read the passage. Only read for the thesis and any specific support of the thesis. You already know that the passage is argumentative, possibly from looking over the text, as well as looking at the nature of the questions. Notice that the passage does not have any bibliographical information, so you need to rely on looking for the thesis and the main ideas in order to give the passage a brief title. Remember: the thesis is often, but not always, contained in the first paragraph.

MCAT Comprehension Review Exercise

The United States school system is in crisis. As middle-class families continue to move out of the city into the suburbs, the gap between the education of the rich and the poor continues to grow wider. Wealthy families have always had more options available to them than poor families. While a lack of financial resources leaves children of poor families trapped in inner-city schools, money has allowed the children of wealthy families to enroll in private schools or to live in expensive houses in "good" public school districts.

"What is to be done" about the current state of the public school system has been a topic of debate for more than 50 years. Recently, failure to compete in international technological markets and an upcoming Presidential election have heightened the intensity of this debate. Conservatives have proposed a new plan called "Choice" that would operate on the model of the free market.

As the system now stands, the number of students per public school, largely determined by city districts, dictates the allocation of government funds in public schools. Choice would turn the United States school system into a mix of public, private, and parochial schools competing with one another for students and for government funding. By supplementing student tuition at private institutions, Choice would open private schools to more students. Advocates claim that public schools could then begin to compete with private schools for students. In turn, this competition would force public schools to increase their academic excellence in order to attract students with several schooling options open to them.

Proponents of Choice claim that competition for students, "customers," and for government funding would ensure excellence in schools. Families would be given vouchers to spend at the school, public or private, of their choice. Those in favor of Choice argue that the voucher system would allow families with meager funds to send their children to first-rate private institutions. They also claim that the program would give parents more options in selecting public schools for their children. In most states today, parents must send their children to the public school designated by their housing district. Under the proposed plan, parents would be free to choose the school they would like their children to attend.

Critics of Choice claim that the plan is mostly political rhetoric. Because private schools today are almost entirely full, the Choice plan would necessitate rapid and extensive rebuilding, something the government is not offering to fund. More radical critics of the plan claim that Choice would only make the education of the rich better and the education of the poor worse. They claim that the government will not be able to provide the enormous funds necessary to make private education a real option for all families. Further, with government money all tied up in vouchers that will be inadequate for most, funds will not be available to help inner-city schools rebuild their programs. In a free-market educational system, inner-city schools will never be competitive.

Before a truly "free" market can be opened, public school systems need to be restructured and refinanced. Before spending money on voucher experiments, the government needs to spend money on restructuring public schools.

Type of passage: ______________________________

A working title for this passage: ______________________________

Summarize the main topic of this passage in one sentence.

____

Using brief phrases, summarize the main support for each paragraph.

....

....

....

....

....

....

What is the actual thesis of the passage?

____

Discussion of the MCAT Comprehension Review Exercise

Notice that the thesis of this passage is in the last paragraph. Allow yourself to be flexible when it comes to finding the thesis in a passage—in general, you can find the thesis at the beginning.

Also notice that in this particular argument, the author includes viewpoints from both sides of the debate, not just one. However, the argument is not simply reporting on both sides and then leaving it up to the reader to judge the debate; this passage definitely contains an opinion about voucher experiments in schooling, even after reporting on both sides of the argument.

Overall, learn to look at MCAT passages as a whole for main ideas and context. Learn to quickly assess passages before reading them more carefully; in doing so, you will work more efficiently and effectively.

Ask yourself these questions for each passage that you read for better comprehension:

1. What is the purpose of this passage?
2. What is the thesis of the passage?
3. What is a brief title I can give this passage?
4. What are the main points of each paragraph?

Now practice the technique of skimming for the main idea in a practice MCAT passage.

Directions:
Give yourself 9 minutes to read this passage and answer the questions that follow. This is how much time you would have on a real MCAT Verbal Reasoning passage. Record the times that you start and finish reading this passage in minutes and seconds. Subtract your starting time from your finishing time to find your total.

MCAT Practice Passage IV

	Minutes	Seconds	
Your finishing time:			
Your starting time:			(subtract)
Your total time:			

Write starting time now, and begin reading.

MCAT Practice Passage IV

Logging is encroaching on the rain forest in the state of Sarawak on the island of Borneo. Sarawak is in the northwest of Borneo, and rain forest occupies most of Sarawak's nearly 50,000 square miles. Borneo's rain forest currently contains 20,000 species of trees, hundreds of species of butterflies, 180 species of mammals, and over 100 kinds of fruiting trees, but logging is threatening the diversity of species. In addition, 24 ethnic groups dwell in the forests, most employing primitive agriculture but some depending on hunting and gathering in the forest to survive. The effects of logging threaten not only the lifestyles but the very lives of these nomadic people.

The loggers argue that their methods are actually more beneficial to the rain forest than the agricultural techniques of the native farmers. However, although the loggers cut select trees rather than clear-cutting the forest, even this method causes a great deal of damage. Bulldozers cut roads through the growth randomly, sometimes along the crests and sides of hills. This causes erosion during the daily rains, therefore polluting streams and making reseeding impossible. Each felled tree hits or topples up to 10 more when it falls. Separate crews go through the forest to clear away the cut trees, causing even more disruption.

Bulldozers have indiscriminately cut their roads and logging camps out of families' rice farms, on which the native people formerly employed crop rotation to preserve the land. Roads have even been cut through the burial ground of the Penan people.

The nomadic Penan people use the rain forest for shelter, game, and plants for food. Western-style progress would not be completely without its benefits to these people—few live to the age of 50, and agricultural and medical development has been stultified by religious superstitions. But logging makes the transition to modernity uncomfortable, difficult, and maybe impossible. First, cutting roads and the destruction of removing trees even selectively logged has disrupted the ecologic system—many of the sago palms on which the Penan depend for most of their carbohydrates are gone, and wild game have been driven away. Penan men now have to hunt for days instead of hours to find game to feed their families, and sometimes their families go hungry. Second, the government has enacted laws against protests and logging. Many Penan protesters have been detained for two weeks or more, and are totally baffled by the country's Western court procedures—conducted in English—when their cases come to trial. Logging has taken away their livelihood and has jailed and terrorized them for their attempts to get it back.

The worst heartbreak is that the high quality, ancient hardwood from the rainforest is not being used, as it could be, for homes, or by master woodworkers for fine furniture. It is being turned into plywood. Because loggers do not have to pay for property rights, and labor is basically free, the price for Borneo's hardwood trees undercuts that of soft farmed woods, such as pine, that are usually used for plywood. Most of the wood is sold to Japanese companies to make molds for concrete, of which most of their buildings are constructed. These molds can be used up to three times and are then sent to landfills or burned. In these fires, it is the future of the rain forest, and the lifestyles and lives of the native people of Sarawak, that are going up in smoke.

Adapted from L. Rosenthal, *Logging and the Destruction of Penan Lifestyle.* © 1989 by The Journal of Cultural Anthropology.

Word count: 640 (see Chapter 3, How to Compute Reading Rates)

Directions:
Write the time you finished reading in the space provided at the beginning of the passage. Subtract your starting time from your finishing time to find out how long it took you to read it. This is your reading time.

Your reading time for MCAT Practice Passage IV is: ____________________

Remember to ask yourself these questions for each passage that you read for better comprehension:

1. What is the purpose of this passage?
2. What is the thesis of the passage?
3. What is a brief title I can give this passage?
4. What are the main points of each paragraph?

Comprehension Questions

1. Which of the following statements is implied by the passage?

A. Logging in the rain forest threatens diversity of plant species because it threatens the diversity of the inhabitants.

B. Logging in the rain forest threatens the condition of the soil because it threatens the lives of the inhabitants.

C. Logging in the rain forest threatens the lives of the inhabitants because it diminishes the diversity of plant species.

D. Logging in the rain forest threatens Borneo's economy because it threatens the supply of trees to Japan.

2. Which of the following effects are the result of logging in Sarawak?

I. Clear-cutting of forest areas
II. Diminished food supply
III. Soil erosion

A. II only
B. I and II only
C. II and III only
D. I, II, and III

3. Why does the author say the future is "going up in smoke" in the last sentence?

A. The author objects to the burning of industrial waste.
B. The wood fueling the fire represents the Penan people's livelihood.
C. The author advocates only domestic use for rain forest products.
D. Loggers are clear-cutting and burning rain forest land.

4. Which of the following policies would be solutions to the problems cited by the author?

I. Cessation of all logging in Sarawak
II. Paying the Penan people a decent wage for their labor
III. Conducting trials in the Penan's native language

A. I and III only
B. II and III only
C. III only
D. I, II, and III

5. Why do Penan men now have to hunt for days instead of hours?

A. Malnutrition makes them tire more easily.
B. Falling trees have killed many rain forest game animals.
C. Penan families are increasing in size.
D. Rain forest game animals have been killed or frightened by the logging.

6. Why are the Penan people's lives threatened?

A. Dangerous conditions in Sarawak jails
B. Ecologic changes have reduced their food supply
C. Inability to earn enough to pay for shelter
D. Inability to make the transition to modernity

7. Which of the following ideas is implied by the passage?

A. All the rain forest in Borneo is in the state of Sarawak.
B. Sarawak's rain forest covers more than 50,000 square miles.
C. Borneo contains more than one state.
D. Penan is a city in Sarawak.

8. Which of the following results is NOT an effect of logging?

A. Lower wages for Penan workers
B. Disregard for traditional patterns of living
C. Pollution of the water supply
D. Enactment of laws against protests of logging operations

Directions:
Correct your answers by looking at the Answers and Explanations section at the end of this chapter. Allow 12.5 percentage points for each correct answer.

MCAT Practice Passage IV Comprehension Score and Reading Time

Your comprehension test score ________%. *Your reading time* ____________

Discussion of MCAT Practice Passage IV

One of the best clues in the passage is the citation. Note that the citation title refers to the "destruction of Penan lifestyle." This title basically tells you two things: the topic of the passage and the attitude of the author. To title a piece so strongly, the author must be concerned and in favor of the Penan people's right to a native lifestyle. The source of the passage also contains some useful information. This piece appears to come from a social anthropology journal. This tells you that the cultural aspects of the Penan people are the likely focus of the author.

The passage is informative/expository with a biased, argumentative slant. The author clearly appears in favor of the Penan people and repeatedly points out the destructive activities of loggers. Every time a Penan ritual is discussed, the negative influence of logging activities on Penan activities and culture is emphasized. Keep the author's tone in mind when answering the questions.

Answers and Explanations to MCAT Practice Passage IV

1. **C** As you read this passage, remember to make a mental map of the flow of information contained in each paragraph. The first paragraph provides the answer to the first question. The species of plants and animals are discussed in the third sentence, as is the threat to the diversity of these species. By inference, you can support choice C. By decreasing the number of species of plants, you would expect some threat to people dependent on plants and animals for food. Choice A is incorrect because it transposes the correct relationship between plant species and inhabitants. Choice B is wrong because the soil is not emphasized in the passage. Choice D can be eliminated because Borneo's economy is not discussed in the passage.
2. **C** To answer an extended multiple-choice question, remember to evaluate each statement independently. Statement I is not supported because sentence two of the second paragraph states that loggers selectively cut trees rather than clear-cutting forests. Therefore, eliminate choices B and D. Statement II is supported by the fourth paragraph. Statement III is supported by the discussion of erosion in the second paragraph. Thus, choice C is correct.
3. **B** This simple inference question requires you to understand what the passage implies rather than what it specifically states. To answer an inference question correctly, think about the attitudes and

principles discussed in the passage. Draw a conclusion from these principles that matches one of the answer choices. In this passage, the last sentence uses the analogy of burning to describe the destruction of the lives and lifestyle of Sarawak native people. This is supported by choice B. Choices A and D are factual choices that do not describe the life changes of the people. Choice C is not supported by the passage.

4. **A** Evaluate each statement on its own merit. Statement I is supported by the logic presented in the passage. A cessation of logging would be expected to improve the problems cited by the author. This eliminates choices B, C, and D, which do not have statement I as an option. The fourth paragraph states that conducting trials in a way that the native people can comprehend would be expected to be an improvement to the current situation. The issue of wages and their effect on the Penan people is not discussed in the passage.

5. **D** This question is a fact-based question. Remember that fact questions require you to report information that was specifically stated in the passage. It is helpful to go back to the passage to find the information being asked about. If you made a mental map as you read or strategic notes in the margins, it will be easy to find the answers to these questions. The answer is found in the fourth paragraph. The Penan men have to hunt for days instead of hours because the wild game have been driven away by logging and disruption of the ecologic system.

6. **B** Use the process of elimination to answer this question. Choice A is not a supported statement because jail conditions are not discussed. Choice B is a true statement, supported by many parts of the passage. Choice C is not supported because paragraph four states that the Penan people use the rain forest for shelter. Choice D is more difficult. It is true that the Penan people are not a modern civilization. However, to decide whether choice B or D better addresses the question and the passage as a whole, think about the author's tone and bias. Is the problem that the loggers are impinging on the Penan people, or are the Penan people not going with the flow of modern times? The passage stresses the effects of the loggers on the native people. The ecologic changes leading to real threats to the Penan people are stressed, so choice B is the best choice.

7. **C** Evaluate each choice based on its own merit. Choice A is not supported because Sarawak is contained in Borneo and is occupied primarily by rain forest. It is never implied that all the rain forest in Borneo is in the state of Sarawak. The passage states that rain forest contains most of Sarawak's 50,000 square miles. Sarawak does not cover more than 50,000 square miles. Choice D is incorrect because the Penan are described as a native nomadic people of the rain forest. Choice C is the best choice based on the process of elimination. In addition, the first sentence of the first paragraph introduces Sarawak as a northwest state of Borneo. This implies that there may be other states.

8. **A** Choices B, C, and D are supported throughout the passage as effects of logging. Wages for Penan laborers are not discussed. The third sentence of the final paragraph even suggests that the labor for logging is basically free.

Chapter 5

Using Key Words to Read and Comprehend

What Are Key Words?

Key words are the **essential words** or the words without which the meaning of the sentence would be lost. In the sentence, "Brisk exercise several times a week can be good for you, whether it be swimming, biking, or running," the key words are **brisk, exercise, good, swimming, biking,** and **running.** Marking key words is particularly helpful when reading passages for the MCAT Verbal Reasoning section because the key words in the passage might also be key words in the questions. When you are aware of these words, you may more easily link what you read to the correct answer.

For example, read this sentence: The speed of light has now been determined to be 186,000 miles per second. The sentence would read much more quickly if it were written as: Light's speed = 186,000 mps.

The following paragraph is from a practice MCAT passage you have already read. Key words have been marked in bold. First, read through the paragraph to understand why each word has been bolded. Next, read the passage again, focusing **only** on the **highlighted** words.

The **United States public school system** is in crisis. As **middle-class families** continue to move out of the **city into** the **suburbs,** the **gap** between the **education** of the **rich** and the **poor** continues to **grow** wider. **Wealthy families** have always had **more options** available to them than **poor families.** While a **lack** of **financial resources** leaves **children** of **poor families** trapped in **inner-city schools,** money has allowed the **children** of **wealthy families** to enroll in **private schools,** or to live in **expensive houses** in "good" **public school** districts.

The words "United States public school system" were highlighted because they are the main topic or framework in which we place the paragraph. The next key words, when grouped together, read "middle-class families city into suburbs," which provides us with a subject and a direction—we see briefly where middle-class families are going. The next grouping of words reads, "gap education rich poor grow," which, if we quickly rearrange for clarity, would read, "education gap rich poor grow(s)." The next grouping of words reads, "Wealthy families more options poor families," a fairly clear meaning. If you continue reading the key words, the main idea of this paragraph is understood quickly.

Using Key Words for Better Comprehension

Key words help you read faster with greater comprehension. These words allow you to read at a greater speed by encouraging selectivity in your reading. In this chapter, we will focus on how to identify what key words are important in the passage and question stems. Skimming and scanning techniques using key words will be discussed in Chapter 6.

There is no formula to identify key words and phrases. You need to develop your own system as a reader for singling out key words within paragraphs. However, here are some useful tips:

1. Look for the **bigger words**—proper nouns, active verbs that have a **direct bearing** on the meaning of the passage.
2. Look for words that **catch your eye immediately** as being important to the direct meaning of a sentence.

If you soften your focus on a paragraph or passage to see only the key words, it should take you less time to get an idea of what the paragraph is about. Do not worry about reading the filler words; these words will be filled in by your mind automatically through association.

Using Key Words to Read Passages

When you first read an MCAT passage, quickly skim it first to get the gist of what the passage is about. Then, read for key words. Again, it is a good idea to practice reading for key words as much as you can. When you practice, use a pencil to quickly underline key words, then read back over the passage reading only these words. You will get in the habit of looking for key words, so that soon you will be able to note these words mentally without having to use your pencil.

Key-Word Exercise 1

Directions:
Two copies of the same paragraph are given below. Quickly skim the first paragraph. Then, reread the paragraph, using your pencil to mark any key words. A second copy of the paragraph follows with possible key words marked for your reference.

A dwarf star is a star with a relatively small diameter. Because of their small size, dwarf stars do not appear very bright. The sun is an average-size star, and dwarf stars have diameters less than that of the sun. There are two different types of dwarf star, distinguished by their color. Red dwarfs are cooler than the sun. They are the most common type of star in the sky and seem to be scaled-down versions of ordinary stars like the sun. White dwarfs are much hotter—white hot, in fact. They may be twice the temperature of the sun. Although a white dwarf contains as much matter as the sun, this mass is condensed into a sphere the size of a planet. Therefore, white dwarf stars are very dense, and a thimbleful of white dwarf material would weigh many tons. White dwarfs are thought to represent the final stages of a star's life, when it has collapsed and is fading away. After several hundred million years, a white dwarf will have cooled off so that it ceases to shine. In this invisible state, it is called a black dwarf.

Shown below is the paragraph with possible key words highlighted. Compare this with your version. Remember that everyone finds their own key words—whatever words are important to get the general meaning of the sentence.

Possible Key-Word Marking
A **dwarf star** is a star with a relatively **small diameter.** Because of their small size, dwarf stars do **not** appear very **bright.** The **sun** is an **average-size** star, and **dwarf stars** have **diameters less than** that of the sun. There are **two** different **types** of dwarf star, **distinguished by** their **color. Red dwarfs** are **cooler than** the **sun.** They are the **most common** type of star in the sky and seem to be **scaled-down** versions of **ordinary stars** like the sun. **White**

dwarfs are much **hotter**—white hot, in fact. They may be **twice** the **temperature** of the **sun.** Although a **white dwarf contains as much matter as** the **sun,** this **mass** is **condensed** into a **sphere** the **size** of a **planet.** Therefore, **white dwarf** stars are very **dense,** and a **thimbleful** of white dwarf **material** would **weigh** many **tons.** White dwarfs are thought to **represent** the **final stages** of a **star's life,** when it has **collapsed** and is **fading** away. **After several hundred million years,** a **white dwarf** will have **cooled** off so that it **ceases to shine.** In this **invisible** state, it is **called** a **black dwarf.**

Directions:
Go back and read your marked paragraph again, reading only the key words, and compare them to the key words marked in this paragraph. By practicing this technique, you should be able to train your eyes to read only the most essential information, stripping away all other words and phrases that are not absolutely essential to understand the paragraph.

Key-Word Exercise 2

Directions:
Two copies of the same paragraph are given below. Quickly skim the first paragraph. Then reread the paragraph, using your pencil to mark any key words. A second copy of the paragraph follows with possible key words marked for your reference.

From a strictly biological standpoint, disease and dysfunction have a strong natural basis. On a planet with limited natural resources such as ours, overpopulation can lead to chronic shortages and intense stress on the biosphere. Death and disease, as much as they are feared, serve as natural balances to the forces of birth and growth. In a Darwinian sense, scourges like cancer and AIDS serve important functions in our continuing evolution. Periodic, pandemic outbreaks of disease weed out the least viable in the population. What is left is a smaller but stronger population. The more we attempt to delay and eliminate such important population checks, the more we endanger the safety of future generations. Nevertheless, as a civilized race, we take pride in the very fact that we have overcome the savage side of our natural existence. Eliminating pain and suffering has become a fixation, and we try everything possible to remove them from our lives. At the same time, we ignore their vital biological significance.

Possible Key-Word Marking
From a strictly **biological** standpoint, **disease** and **dysfunction** have a **strong natural basis.** On a planet with **limited** natural **resources** such as ours, **overpopulation** can lead to chronic **shortages** and intense **stress** on the biosphere. **Death** and **disease,** as much as they are feared, serve as **natural balances** to the forces of birth and growth. In a **Darwinian** sense, scourges like **cancer** and **AIDS** serve **important functions** in our continuing evolution. Periodic, pandemic **outbreaks of disease weed out** the **least viable** in the population. What is left is a **smaller but stronger population.** The more we attempt to **delay** and **eliminate** such important **population checks,** the more we **endanger** the **safety** of future generations. Nevertheless, as a **civilized** race, we take pride in the very fact that we have **overcome** the

savage side of our natural existence. **Eliminating pain and suffering** has become a **fixation,** and we try everything possible to remove them from our lives. At the same time, **we ignore** their **vital biological significance.**

Directions:
Go back and read your marked paragraph again, reading only the key words, and compare it to the key words marked in this paragraph. You know that you have marked appropriate key words when you can still get the importance of a paragraph or passage by just reading the key words.

Using Key Words to Skim Question Stems

A second way to use key words on the MCAT Verbal Reasoning section is to underline them as you skim the question stems. Keep in mind that many of the question stems contain key words or phrases. If a question stem does not contain key words or phrases, it is often less useful in helping you identify potential answers when you read the text.

Below are some questions similar to recent MCAT Verbal Reasoning questions. Look at the sentences and determine which contain key words or phrases.

Stem 1: According to the passage, the invention of nuclear weapons has:
Key words and phrases include **invention** and **nuclear weapons.**

Stem 2: The passage suggests that destruction of the wilderness has NOT been accompanied by the:
Key words and phrases include **destruction, wilderness, NOT,** and **accompanied.**

Stem 3: Which of the following ideas would most challenge the author's conception of culture as revealed in the passage?
Key words and phrases include **ideas, challenge, conception,** and **culture.**

Question-Stem Exercise

For the following five sample Verbal Reasoning question stems, quickly skim each and underline key words and phrases. Possible answers follow the question stems.

1. According to the passage, which of the following is true of a satisfactory explanation of how a complex entity like a language works?
2. Based on information given in the passage, the types of components of the diurnal precipitation cycle are:
3. What does the passage propose about strategies that combine patterns of "natural" powers with "acquired" powers?
4. The author's conclusions would be most challenged by which of the following?
5. Based on information provided in the passage, with which of the following would the author most likely agree?

Possible Key Words and Phases

1. Explanation, complex entity, language, works
2. Components, diurnal precipitation cycle

3. Strategies, combine, "natural," "acquired," powers
4. Conclusions, most challenged
5. Which, author, agree

Remember that question-stem reading is only part of the overall strategy. You will probably find it strategic to first skim the question stems for 15–20 seconds. Then, skim the passage topic sentences for key words to gain an idea of the passage. Finally, begin a full attack on carefully reading the passage.

The best way to get the hang of reading for key words is to practice. Now, let's try another MCAT sample passage. Use your pencil as you read through this MCAT passage, and mark all the key words. Then, read the passage again, only reading the key words. Time yourself for the first and the second reading to see if there is a difference.

At the end of the chapter, you will find a copy of this passage with possible key words marked. After you finish reading and answering the questions, compare the two versions of the passage.

Directions:
Record the times that you start and finish marking and reading this passage in minutes and seconds. Subtract your starting time from your finishing time to find your total. Give yourself a total of 9 minutes to read the passage and answer the questions.

MCAT Practice Passage V

Marking key words	Minutes	Seconds
Your finishing time:		
Your starting time:		(subtract)
Your total time:		

Reading only marked key words	Minutes	Seconds
Your finishing time:		
Your starting time:		(subtract)
Your total time:		

Write starting time now, and begin reading.

MCAT Practice Passage V

Biblical scholars have long debated the meaning behind the seemingly contradictory depictions of the relationship between God and Abraham in Genesis 18 and Genesis 22. Although a tension may exist between the Abraham of Genesis 18:22–23 and the Abraham of Genesis 22, the two are certainly not irreconcilable. The Abraham of Genesis 18 does not challenge the faithfulness of the Abraham of Genesis 22 because the two chapters present Abraham relating to the Lord in two very different situations. The first scene is a lesson in justice, whereas the second is a test of faith. Taken together, the two scenes present a relationship between man and God in which man may question God concerning the nature of justice, provided he does not question the Lord in matters concerning faith. Both interactions point to a hierarchical relationship between Abraham and the Lord, one in which Abraham pleases the Lord as long as he acknowledges and respects the Lord's ultimate, overriding power.

In Genesis 18, Abraham successfully questions the Lord without angering him. Abraham does not arouse the wrath of God because his manner in addressing the Lord remains humble at all times. Abraham begins most of his questions with "Oh let not the Lord be angry . . .," and states repeatedly: "Behold, I have taken upon myself to speak to the Lord, I who am but dust and ashes." One can see that while Abraham may question the Lord, he also reaffirms the Lord's greater power and his own mental inferiority.

The Lord does not ask Abraham to perform any task in Genesis 18. In this interaction, the Lord merely tells Abraham of his plan to destroy Sodom and Gomorrah and almost invited questions by telling Abraham: "Shall I hide from Abraham what I am about to do, seeing that Abraham shall become a great and mighty nation, and all the nations of the earth shall bless themselves by him? No, for I have chosen him, that he may charge his children and his household after him to keep the way of the Lord by doing righteousness and justice . . ." (Genesis 18:17). Thus, Abraham's questions to the Lord do not arise out of insolence, but out of a desire to understand the nature of the Lord's justice, which Abraham and his descendants have been commanded to uphold.

In Genesis 22, the interaction between the Lord and Abraham takes place on quite different terms from those of Genesis 18. In this later chapter, the Lord directly asks Abraham to perform a task for him. He tests Abraham's faith, telling him to sacrifice his innocent son, a command most would find cruelly unjust. However, because he has been directly called upon to act by the Lord, Abraham cannot protest this injustice. Any misgivings or qualms on Abraham's part would dignify great insolence and a lack of respect for the power of the Lord. Thus, in order to demonstrate his understanding of the hierarchical nature of the relationship between himself and the Lord, Abraham obeys the Lord without hesitation.

Taken together, Genesis 18 and 22 describe a clearly unequal relationship between Abraham and the Lord, one in which Abraham must at all times respect the superior position of the Lord. Abraham is permitted to question the Lord in matters concerning the nature of justice, but only when his own action is not involved. When Abraham himself is called upon to act by the Lord, he must obey without hesitation. Questioning a command from the Lord would undermine the hierarchy of their relationship. Thus, because he understands the nature of his relationship to the Lord, Abraham remains a faithful servant to him at all times, questioning the essence of God's justice only when appropriate according to the terms of their relationship.

Word Count: 689

Directions:
Record the time you finished marking and reading in the space provided at the beginning of the passage. Subtract your starting time from your finishing time to find out how long it took you to read it. Then, figure your reading rate.

Your reading rate is: ______________________

Comprehension Questions

Answer the following questions from memory or from referring back to the passage. Try to answer all the questions in 5 minutes or less.

1. In Genesis 22, Abraham follows God's commands:

A. in order to please God.
B. in order to please his worth to God.
C. because he respects God.
D. because he is inferior to God.

2. The one thing Abraham can never do is:

A. anger God.
B. question God.
C. disobey God.
D. displease God.

3. The author of this passage believes that the Bible is:

A. confusing.
B. intriguing.
C. compelling.
D. consistent.

4. In Genesis 22, God tests Abraham:

A. to make sure that Abraham understands his role.
B. because God does not trust Abraham.
C. because God is angry with Abraham.
D. to further illustrate God's systems of punishment.

5. From the passage, the reader can infer that God is:

A. amiable.
B. wrathful.
C. indecisive.
D. reasonable.

6. Abraham can question God when:

A. he does not understand God's actions.
B. he does not understand God's instructions.
C. God wants him to ask questions.
D. he does not like God's actions.

7. The relationship of God to Abraham is most like that of a:

A. doctor to patient.
B. manager to employee.
C. husband to wife.
D. pope to king.

8. From the passage, it is clear that Abraham:

A. fears God.
B. trusts God.
C. loves God.
D. likes God.

Directions:
Correct your answers by using the Answers and Explanations section. Allow 12.5 percentage points for each correct answer.

MCAT Practice Passage V Comprehension Score and Reading Time

Your comprehension test score ________*%. Your reading rate (find on rate table)* ____________.

Discussion of MCAT Practice Passage V

This passage has an argument, and it is expository. It explains one way of reading the Bible and the relationship between the Lord and Abraham, but because there are many ways of reading the Bible, this passage is attempting to convince readers to interpret the Bible in a particular way. Notice that there is no citation for this passage to give important clues.

In a complex passage like this, it is important to make a mental map of the coverage of each paragraph and small notations in the margins. Mapping the paragraphs should include a thesis and evidence to support that thesis. The first paragraph contains the thesis by presenting the argument that a hierarchical relationship exists between God and Abraham, as shown in Genesis 18 and 22. Genesis 18 is a lesson in justice, and Genesis 22 is a lesson in faith. The rest of the paragraphs give evidence for this argument. The second paragraph discusses Genesis 18; although Abraham questions God, he also does so respectfully and humbly. In the third paragraph, God invites questions of Abraham, but only out of a desire to understand the Lord's justice. Paragraph four discusses Genesis 22, in which God asks Abraham to perform a task—sacrificing his innocent son. The fifth paragraph compares God's and Abraham's relationship as portrayed in Genesis 18 and 22.

Answers and Explanations to MCAT Practice Passage V

1. **D** This passage explicitly argues that the relationship of God to Abraham is a hierarchical one, in which Abraham is clearly permitted to question God but is never permitted to disobey him. Paragraph four clearly points out that in Genesis 22, Abraham demonstrates his understanding of the hierarchical relationship.
2. **C** Choice B is incorrect because the passage states that Abraham may question God. However, in the second paragraph, the passage does imply that Abraham is careful not to arouse the wrath of God when questioning him. The passage does not specifically mention whether it is permitted for Abraham to displease or anger God, but it is clear that he is never permitted to disobey him. Choice C is well supported in paragraphs four and five.
3. **D** Remember that thesis statements frequently are found at the end of the first paragraph. In this passage, this is the case. Note that the last sentence of the first paragraph emphasizes the consistency of Genesis 18 and Genesis 22. This is the author's primary underlying claim.

4. **A** Check your margin notations or mental map to see which paragraph contains information on Genesis 22. In the fourth paragraph, God essentially is training Abraham for his future role.
5. **B** The second paragraph uses the term "wrath of God." This sets the tone for the rest of the passage and explains the care with which Abraham communicates and interacts with God. The other choices are not as well supported. Choice A implies friendliness. There is no evidence of friendly interaction between Abraham and God. The passage does not give any indication that God is indecisive. No discussion is offered about the reasonableness of God.
6. **C** This is a relatively difficult question. Abraham can question God in matters concerning the nature of justice. He can also question God when God wants to be questioned. Note how Abraham carefully and humbly words all questions to remain subordinate. Choice D is incorrect because it is not important whether or not Abraham likes God's actions. Choices A and B are not as good as choice C. Abraham is invited to question God. Abraham may not question God for lack of understanding.
7. **B** This is an example of an application question. This question asks for you to make an analogy of the relationship between God and Abraham, and apply it to the answer choices. Notice that the passage makes a clear hierarchical relationship between God and Abraham. This relationship is most like a manager to an employee.
8. **A** Be careful not to interject your feelings for God when answering this question! Just answer the question based on what you can support from the passage. In the second paragraph, Abraham's fear of God is clear when he questions God.

MCAT Practice Passage V: Key Words and Phrases

Biblical scholars have long **debated** the **meaning** behind the **seemingly contradictory depictions** of the **relationship** between **God** and **Abraham** in **Genesis 18** and **Genesis 22.** Although a **tension may exist between** the **Abraham** of **Genesis 18:22–23** and the **Abraham of Genesis 22,** the **two** are certainly **not irreconcilable.** The Abraham of **Genesis 18** does **not challenge** the **faithfulness** of the Abraham of **Genesis 22** because the two chapters present **Abraham relating** to the **Lord** in two very **different situations.** The **first** scene is a **lesson** in **justice,** whereas the **second** is a **test** of **faith.** Taken **together,** the **two** scenes **present** a **relationship** between man and God in which **man** may **question God concerning** the nature of **justice, provided** he does **not question** the **Lord** in matters concerning **faith.** Both interactions point to a **hierarchical relationship** between **Abraham** and the **Lord,** one in which **Abraham pleases** the **Lord** as long as he **acknowledges** and **respects** the **Lord's** ultimate, overriding **power.**

In **Genesis 18, Abraham** successfully **questions** the **Lord without angering him.** Abraham does not arouse the wrath of God because his **manner** in addressing the Lord **remains humble** at all times. Abraham **begins** most of his **questions** with **"Oh let not the Lord be angry . . .,"** and **states** repeatedly: **"Behold, I have taken upon myself to speak to the Lord, I who am but dust and ashes."** One can see that while **Abraham** may question the Lord, he also **reaffirms** the **Lord's** greater **power** and his **own mental inferiority.**

The **Lord** does **not ask Abraham** to **perform** any **task** in **Genesis 18.** In this interaction, the **Lord** merely **tells Abraham** of his **plan** to **destroy Sodom** and **Gomorrah,** and almost **invites questions** by telling Abraham: **"Shall I hide from Abraham what I am about to do, seeing that Abraham shall become a great and mighty nation, and all the nations of the earth shall bless themselves by him? No, for I have chosen him, that he may charge his children and his household after him to keep the way of the Lord by doing righteousness and justice . . ." (Genesis 18:17).** Thus, Abraham's **questions** to the Lord do **not arise** out of **insolence,** but out of a **desire** to **understand** the nature of the **Lord's justice,** which

Abraham and his descendants have been commanded to uphold.

In **Genesis 22,** the **interaction** between the Lord and Abraham takes place on quite **different terms** from those of **Genesis 18.** In this later chapter, the **Lord** directly **asks Abraham** to **perform** a **task** for him. He **tests Abraham's faith,** telling him to **sacrifice** his **innocent son,** a command most would find cruelly unjust. However, **because** he has been **directly called upon** to act by the **Lord, Abraham cannot protest** this injustice. Any **misgivings** or **qualms** on Abraham's part would **signify** great **insolence** and a **lack of respect** for the power of the **Lord.** Thus, in order to **demonstrate** his understanding of the **hierarchical** nature of the **relationship** between himself and the Lord, **Abraham obeys** the Lord without hesitation.

Taken together, **Genesis 18 and 22 describe** a clearly **unequal relationship** between Abraham and the Lord, one in which **Abraham** must at all times **respect** the **superior position** of the **Lord.** Abraham is permitted to question the Lord in matters concerning the nature of justice, but only when his own action is not involved. When Abraham himself is called upon to act by the Lord, he must obey without hesitation. Questioning a command from the Lord would undermine the hierarchy of their relationship. Thus, because he understands the nature of his relationship to the Lord, **Abraham** remains a **faithful servant** to him at all times, **questioning** the essence of **God's justice** only **when appropriate** according **to** the **terms** of their **relationship.**

Chapter 6

Skimming, Scanning, and Marking Text

Skimming and scanning are reading techniques that you probably use every day. By using them more consciously, you can increase both your reading comprehension and your ability to locate information in a passage. Both of these skills are particularly important when reading MCAT passages and answering questions.

Skimming

Skimming involves going over a text more quickly than your normal reading rate for the purpose of **understanding only the main idea** without the details. Many people use this technique when studying. For example, when taking notes from reading material, you probably skim through material to find the important information. When studying, you may use skimming to see ahead of time what the general idea of a text is, so that when you read more carefully, the details will fall into place in a way that is easier to remember.

When you skim, try to **anticipate** and **predict** what the passage is about based on the important **key words** and **phrases.** Key words carry important meaning.

Skimming Drill 1

Below are some words and phrases from an article. See if you can anticipate what this article will be about, based on these few words or phrases.

professor
Institute of Biochemistry
hard-working man
results of experiments
published
confession
invention
different results
fraud
regrets it

Can you guess, from these few words, what the article is about? See which sentence best summarizes the words listed.

A. A well-known professor who has just published his confessions
B. A scientist who has admitted inventing the results of his experiments
C. A scientist who killed himself because he couldn't get the same results as everybody else
D. A scientist who regrets the publication of the results of his experiments

These key words and phrases probably center around a hard-working professor at an Institute of Biochemistry who may have published some scientific results that he regrets. There may be fraud involved. Which choice fits best? If you guessed choice B, you are correct. This exercise should give you a good idea how useful skimming can be.

Here is another collection of key words and phrases. Determine which choice given below is the best thesis for the passage that contains these words and phrases.

communication
patient relationship
lack of understanding
thought processes
resistance
healing thwarted
belief system
healing
Western medicine
faith
different culture

A. Doctors need training in folk medicine.
B. Medical schools need to train doctors to be better "mechanics."
C. Doctors should spend less time learning about diseases.
D. Doctors are not sufficiently trained in psychology and cultural sensitivity.

These key words and phrases seem to tie together communication problems and patient relationships in medicine. Perhaps there are belief system differences among patients and doctors from different cultures. Words such as "healing thwarted" and "resistance" cause you to wonder if conflict is involved. The best thesis for these words and phrases is choice D.

Skimming Drill 2

Skim this paragraph for main ideas only, then write the main idea in one sentence below the paragraph. Try to come up with a title for the paragraph.

Today, we use science for many different reasons. We use science to get a space shuttle into space, we have saved lives through science by way of artificial organs, the food we eat and the drugs we take every day are products of science. In the eighteenth century, science was hardly so accessible or so widely used. In the novel *Frankenstein*, by Mary Shelley, Victor Frankenstein is curious about what life is all about and how life originated. This curiosity starts early in his life and torments him, ultimately bringing him to his death. Not only curiosity brings him practically to insanity, but also this great desire to control nature and the "physical secrets of the world."

Quick!

Main idea? ____

Title? ____

The main idea in this paragraph has to do with scientific curiosity and the need to control, as it is shown in the character of Victor Frankenstein in the novel *Frankenstein.* A title could be "Scientific Curiosity and Control in *Frankenstein*."

Now, skim the following paragraph:

Being a teacher in Victorian England was at one time thought of as the most enticing, fulfilling career a single woman could possibly pursue. Education was a popular choice of profession for middle-class women from the mid-nineteenth through the early twentieth centuries. Traditional feminine tasks, such as the care and education of children within the home, had moved slowly outside the home in keeping with the trends of early industrial England and the expansion of the market economy. Schools increased in number, providing employment opportunities for single women. These opportunities to become teachers "were perceived by the Victorians as 'safe' and quasi–household-centered work that did not jeopardize the single woman's future life as wife and mother." So a new and seemingly simple vocational path was paved for women to become teachers.

Quick!

Main idea? ____

Title? ____

The main idea in this paragraph is that in Victorian England, teaching became a desirable profession for single women. A possible title could be "Teaching: the Emergence of a Profession for Single Victorian Women." Titling can put the passage or paragraph into context and help you to know what information to look for when you are answering questions on the MCAT.

Use skimming when you need to run your eyes over a passage to get a general idea of a writing. This can be the first step you take when you look at an MCAT passage. Skimming will give you a general context for the passage; and from this framework, you can give the passage a title.

Practice skimming by reading newspaper articles very quickly, then attempting to explain to yourself or someone else what the article was about. Or you can skim the article, then put it down and write in a few sentences what you think the article is about.

Scanning

Scanning involves going over a text at a rate that exceeds your normal reading rate. Your intent is different from skimming because you are looking for **specific information** in the text. Look for the definite word, phrase, or idea that you need. For instance, when you are reading MCAT passages and answering questions, scanning comes in handy if you are looking for a key word in a passage that you also saw in a question. You use scanning techniques when you look for a particular name in a phone book or a particular word in the dictionary. You look over the other names or words in order to find exactly what you need.

Try these drills to hone your scanning. You will need a pencil and a watch with a second hand or a timer.

Scanning Drill 1

Directions:
Circle the word that means **almost the same** as the first word in each line. Go as fast as you can, timing yourself. See if you can do all of these in 90 seconds.

1.	stare	gab gale galley gawk gentle garb
2.	little	tin tiny tie tidbit tight tinge tickle
3.	dull	stuff submit stop stoop stupid stocky
4.	cord	romp role rooms root rouge rope
5.	chance	forward fortune frame form forego fraction
6.	plea	appeal ascertain arrant art arrival arrest
7.	amble	wallet ward wane wall wag walk
8.	wait	being behind bide bed beckon begin
9.	divide	part plate pledge plenty pleasure partner
10.	group	gag nag lag gang gall gal gallery
11.	jump	loom loop loose lank lamp leap leer
12.	enjoy	level leech latch lack like lake lever
13.	fat	stout station static stale staunch stuck
14.	unique	organize origin original opposite opulent organ
15.	character	near nature neckwear nausea neat necessity
16.	surplus	respite resolution resolved remaining resign
17.	correct	truck true trim trek trellis treatise tremor
18.	value	wind whine why will work worth widen
19.	evil	wig wily wicked wide widen waken worthy
20.	energy	violence venture verbal vigor veneer vessel
21.	mind	clan plan plain brain please brine clime slime
22.	tan	bag beg beige bear bearing beat beast buckle
23.	bay	golf gulf glut gulch grouch couch hutch
24.	room	character chance channel champagne chamber
25.	dispel	scat scuttle scatter scared scar car care

Time ______________

The answers are at the end of the chapter.

Scanning Drill 2

Directions:
Circle the word that means the **opposite** of the first word in each line. Go as fast as you can, timing yourself as you did for the first drill. See if you can do these all in 90 seconds.

1.	rough	ragged raging sage smooth smell small
2.	dirty	clear clean cling claim clam clumsy calm
3.	finger	finish famished tarnish tingle toe top tap
4.	ceiling	floor flood flute flop flip flue blue flub
5.	casual	dismal normal formal fortunate fortitude fatuous
6.	day	naught narrow naughty night nickel never nuts
7.	alive	dazed dazzled double deceased depressed deed
8.	happy	miserable miserly masterful mink muddy mopped
9.	silly	sailing sinful solemn sapped sunny safe
10.	wonderful	awl anvil apple ant anatomy ask awful
11.	awake	slippery slap slush slim sleeping weeping
12.	dark	late light last lint loft left lift laugh
13.	little	bag bug beg bog hog huge hag hug
14.	icy	hat hit hot cot got gold fold hold
15.	wealth	walking waiting parting poverty paltry
16.	dismal	chair chore cheerful chase chaise chafe
17.	sweet	sweat swindle wine sour spine
18.	laugh	care car carry cry try tray tarry tar
19.	cautious	careful colorful careless careworn candy
20.	go	step staple stipple stop stump stupid steps
21.	stale	frigid fragile frost frantic fresh frump
22.	lazy	easy evil every energetic engine eat
23.	always	niece nimble noise nice never nuts
24.	end	beg big bargain beginning between bud
25.	luminous	bull hull gull dull full pull null

Time ________

The answers to these drills are at the end of this chapter.

Use this kind of specific searching when you are looking for a key word or phrase in an MCAT passage, particularly if the word comes from a question. You can practice scanning by predicting and anticipating the kind of information you need. Remember, you are already pretty good at this technique because you practice this skill every time you look up a word in a dictionary or phone book. All you have to do now is apply this skill to the passages on the MCAT!

Marking Text

Marking text allows you to note important parts of the text and helps you identify sentences you may want to come back to for better understanding. Because you are not allowed to use a highlighter on the MCAT, practice using a pencil to make simple, quick marks in the margin as you read. Table 6-1 contains some examples of marks to use.

Table 6-1. Suggested Marking Techniques

* or underline	Single important idea
|	Important sentences or whole paragraphs
✓	Do not understand
?	Question regarding statement
1, 2, 3, 4, etc.	Items in a series

Try these marks, or find marks that are natural and comfortable for you. Keep your pencil poised over the text as you read through MCAT passages to make necessary marks in the passage. This technique helps you locate important ideas and words when trying to answer questions. In addition, when you allow yourself to mark a line or a section, you are **increasing your efficiency** because you can always come back to the section you marked to find important information. You will not have to waste time trying to find the important parts of the passage.

The following example illustrates what a marked text can look like. A brief explanation of why the text was marked this way follows.

Example of Marked Text

The effect of scores on pretest and post-test of multiplication problems depending on * an in-class or after-school help session with varying levels of a reward system was measured in this study. Third grade students who had been judged by their teachers as having math anxiety took the pretest, then went through a one-month help session, each ? session lasting 30 minutes, three times a week. At the end of the month, a post-test was given, identical to the pretest. Help sessions met in class or after school, and students were given no ① reward, a verbal ② reward, a ③ sticker reward, or both ④ verbal and sticker rewards for correct answers to multiplication flash card drills during the help sessions. Mean average difference between pretests and post-tests showed that, although there was not much difference between the groups that met in class or after school, a greater improved score between the pretest and the post-test correlated with the amount of reward a student received for correct answers during the help sessions, suggesting that a reward system based on verbal rewards and small object rewards may increase scores on math tests for students with math anxiety.

In this paragraph, taken from a psychological abstract, the types of rewards were numbered for easy reference (1, 2, 3). The first sentence seemed to be the main question or idea, so the reader marked it with an asterisk (*). The last long sentence contained several ideas and conclusions, so the reader drew a brief line next to that section of the text (|). Also, the reader was not clear on how the teachers judged whether their students had math anxiety, so the reader wrote a question mark (?) next to the line where this idea was introduced but not clear.

Marking a text this way can go much more quickly and efficiently than using a highlighter or underlining. First, making brief marks takes less time. Second, from these distinct marks, you will know **why** you marked that sentence or section, so that when you come back to it later, you'll know what you were thinking when you read it the first time.

When you are studying for the MCAT, try using the following procedure when skimming, scanning, and marking a text.

1. Quickly preview the questions after the passage (just read the question stems).
2. Preview by skimming the entire passage or article.
3. Record starting time.
4. Read and mark text. Be flexible in your reading.
5. Record finish time.
6. Skim the passage, slowing down on marked sections.
7. Answer questions at the end of the passage or article, scanning for key words.
8. Correct answers.

Reading for Detail

Sometimes you need to read slowly and deliberately for detail. When you study new material or read specific instructions, you naturally slow down and pay attention to the details. What is most important is knowing **when** to slow down and when to skim material.

Your work in determining the main idea will help in this kind of detail reading. Follow these steps when looking for details in a particular passage.

1. Find the main idea. You can do this by titling the passage or putting the main idea into your own words.
2. Look specifically for details about that main idea. These details might be material that illustrates the main idea or that focuses in on a particular aspect of the main idea. Think of the main idea together with its supporting examples as a unit.

Directions:
Record the times that you start and finish reading this passage in minutes and seconds. Subtract your starting time from your finishing time to find your total. Try to read the passage and answer the questions in 9 minutes. Practice question-stem skimming, previewing the passage, and marking the text as you work on this passage.

MCAT Practice Passage VI

	Minutes	Seconds	
Your finishing time:			
Your starting time:			(subtract)
Your total time:			

Record starting time now, and begin reading.

MCAT Practice Passage VI

Every year, thousands of families in the United States alone face the devastating loss of a child as a result of Sudden Infant Death Syndrome, or SIDS. The definition of SIDS reflects medical ignorance regarding its causes; an infant or young child is said to have died from SIDS if the death was unexpected in light of the child's medical history and is unexplained by thorough autopsy. Yet SIDS is the leading cause of death for children under 1 year of age; indeed, every year SIDS claims more lives than cancer, pneumonia, heart disease, child abuse, AIDS, cystic fibrosis, and muscular dystrophy combined during the first 14 years of life.

The tragedy of SIDS is underscored by the scars it leaves on the families of its victims. The absence of an adequate explanation for a loss to SIDS disrupts the normal mourning process and can lead to the breakup of a family, as members either suffer debilitating guilt and shame or resort to blaming each other in attempts to make sense of the death. Even parents that weather a SIDS death with relative success may have severe difficulty in continuing to care for their other children. Sadly, the family affected by SIDS rarely recovers in full.

As a growing body of SIDS research has confirmed, SIDS knows no racial or socioeconomic barriers. And until recently, SIDS appeared to strike healthy infants entirely at random. However, very recent data suggest that infants with subtle central nervous system abnormalities may be disposed to SIDS relative to infants without such abnormalities. These subtle neural abnormalities are in turn believed to be the result of complex processes in fetal development, although these processes themselves are as yet poorly understood. These results are consistent with the long-standing working hypothesis that SIDS is caused by abnormalities in the general mechanisms that regulate an infant's respiration, heart rate, and body temperature during sleep. Because the identification of neural abnormalities depends upon a prior characterization of what constitutes their normal operation, much recent SIDS research has focused on understanding neural development in the average infant.

Medical research holds out the hope that someday a screening procedure for SIDS will be developed, leading to a significant decrease in SIDS related deaths. But by all accounts, that day is far off. In the meantime, though, there are a number of measures parents can take to cope with the threat of SIDS. Because there is some indication that what would have been a SIDS death can be prevented if the infant receives prompt attention, perhaps the most important measure one can take is to learn the skills necessary to revive an infant who has stopped breathing or undergone cardiac arrest. Most communities sponsor infant cardiopulmonary resuscitation (or "CPR") programs at a reasonable cost.

Another, albeit more expensive, measure is to install a system for monitoring a sleeping infant's respiration or heart rate. Such systems sound an alarm if respiration or heart rate falls below a certain predetermined level during sleep.

A third measure is to become involved in the SIDS Alliance, a national organization devoted to funding research into the causes of SIDS, making available information about SIDS, and sponsoring programs directed at helping the families of SIDS victims. Although no family can insulate itself entirely from the threat of SIDS, together, through such organizations as the SIDS Alliance, families can bring closer the day when SIDS is no longer a threat.

Adapted from R. Heftel, *The Facts and Tragedies of SIDS*. © 1995 by R. Heftel.

Word Count: 616

Directions:
In the space provided at the beginning of the passage, write the time you finished reading.

Your reading rate is: ______________________.

Comprehension Questions

Answer these questions from memory or by referring to the passage.

1. Information in the passage implies that:

A. parents who learn CPR are better equipped to cope with a SIDS death.
B. parents who learn CPR may be able to prevent a death from SIDS.
C. CPR might be a cure for SIDS.
D. CPR is easy to learn.

2. According to the passage:

A. the majority of infants who die in their first year die from SIDS.
B. the cause of most infant deaths is unknown.
C. in their first year more children die of SIDS than pneumonia.
D. cancer is the cause of very few infant deaths.

3. Which of the following events would NOT count as evidence for the hypothesis that SIDS is caused by abnormalities in the general mechanisms that regulate an infant's respiration, heart rate, and body temperature during sleep?

I. The discovery that SIDS deaths were more common among infants with a history of frequent fevers
II. The discovery that SIDS deaths were more common among infants with developmental abnormalities
III. The discovery that the average infant's normal body temperature varies more than had previously been thought

A. I only
B. I and II only
C. II and III only
D. I and III only

4. According to the passage, which of the following effects is most likely to happen to a family after it loses a member to SIDS?

A. The parents of the family will encounter difficulties in raising their other children.
B. The family will have difficulties but eventually recover completely.
C. The family will become involved with the SIDS Alliance.
D. The family will have a child to replace the child that was lost to SIDS.

5. Which of the following, based on information presented in the passage, is among the central functions of the SIDS Alliance?

A. Conducting research into the causes of SIDS
B. Maintaining accurate records of SIDS deaths
C. Maintaining support services for families affected by SIDS
D. Encouraging research into the causes of SIDS

6. Which of the following statements accurately summarizes the impact that the passage attributes to the "very recent data" mentioned in the third paragraph?

A. SIDS may be caused by abnormalities occurring in fetal development.
B. All infants are at the same risk of dying from SIDS.
C. SIDS is probably caused by abnormalities in the general mechanisms that regulate an infant's respiration, heart rate, and body temperature during sleep.
D. How infants develop normally is not well understood.

7. A good title for this passage would be:

A. "Coping With SIDS."
B. "The Tragedy of SIDS."
C. "Why We Need the SIDS Alliance."
D. "SIDS: Some Promising Research."

8. Which of the following statements does the author offer as a reason for parents of infants to take CPR courses?

A. CPR courses are inexpensive for what you get.
B. Infant monitoring systems are pointless if one does not know CPR.
C. Timely use of CPR may prevent a death from SIDS.
D. CPR skills are valuable in general.

Directions:
Correct your answers by using the Answers and Explanations section. Allow 12.5 percentage points for each correct answer.

MCAT Practice Passage VI Comprehension Score and Reading Rate

Your comprehension test score ________%. *Your reading rate* ____________.

Discussion of MCAT Practice Passage VI

This is an expository passage; notice how factual information is spread throughout the passage. The passage defines SIDS, its effects and causes, and gives some measures of prevention against SIDS. Also, note the citation at the end of the passage. The author titles the piece to include both "facts" and "tragedies." This implies that the author wishes to point out the negative effects of this condition and the sorrow that SIDS can bring upon a family. The first paragraph defines SIDS and gives some facts about the syndrome. Paragraph two discusses how families are affected by SIDS. Paragraph three talks about some possible causes for the syndrome and explains the reasons for these theories. The next three paragraphs discuss ways to work toward preventing SIDS from happening in the first place. Paragraph four talks about learning infant CPR, the fifth paragraph discusses installing a sound system to monitor an infant's heart rate, and paragraph six talks about becoming involved in SIDS Alliance.

Answers and Explanations to MCAT Practice Passage VI

1. **B** Solve this question by the process of elimination. Eliminate choices A, C, and D because the passage does not suggest that parents who learn CPR are better equipped to cope with SIDS death or that CPR is either easy to learn or a cure for SIDS. Choice B is best because the last section of the fourth paragraph suggests that, in some cases, CPR can prevent a SIDS death.
2. **C** The choices in this question manipulate the facts in the passage and make false implications. That SIDS is the leading cause of infant deaths does not imply that the majority of infant deaths are caused by SIDS, nor (by the same token) that the cause of most infant deaths is unknown. The information does imply that more infants die of SIDS in their first year than of any other cause, such as pneumonia. Conversely, it does not imply that cancer is an uncommon cause of death for infants.
3. **C** Evaluate each statement independently, and use the validity of statements to help eliminate incorrect choices. Statement I would count as evidence for the presented hypothesis. The discovery that SIDS deaths were more common among infants with a history of frequent fevers would support the hypothesis described, whereas the discovery either that SIDS was linked with just any developmental abnormality or that normal infant temperature had a wider range than was previously thought would not support that hypothesis specifically.

4. **A** Making a mental map of this passage aids in finding the answer to this question. Again, use the process of elimination to sift through the answer choices. Paragraph two discusses the implications of a SIDS-related death on the family. The passage states that SIDS-affected families rarely, if ever, recover. The passage does not discuss the likelihood that a SIDS-affected family will become involved with the SIDS Alliance or have another child. It does mention, however, a likelihood that problems will arise with the raising of any remaining children.
5. **C** This is a fact question about the SIDS Alliance, which is discussed in the final paragraph. The SIDS Alliance is not described as actually doing or encouraging SIDS-related research but only funding it. The passage does not mention maintaining accurate records, but it does mention the maintenance of support services for families of SIDS victims.
6. **A** This is a main idea question that asks you to summarize a component of the passage. To answer main idea questions correctly, review the corresponding section of the passage, and organize the facts presented into the basic principles of the text. Draw appropriate conclusions regarding the relationship or importance of the principles to each other. Finally, determine the central thought of the passage based on the relative importance of the principles contained in the passage. For this question, the "very recent data" mentioned in the third paragraph links SIDS to neural abnormalities arising from development. This is a means to discriminate risks among infants. Although the passage asserts that infant development is not well understood, the new evidence does not rely on this assertion.
7. **B** This is also a main idea question. You should look for an overall theme of the passage. The citation at the end of the passage gives you some good clues. The passage is really about SIDS-related facts and the tragedy of SIDS. The best choice is B. The passage addresses coping with SIDS, the SIDS Alliance, and new results in SIDS research in a general context that emphasizes that SIDS is a tragedy.
8. **C** The fourth paragraph addresses this topic. Although each of the alternatives may be offered as a reason to take a CPR class, the passage mentions only the effectiveness that CPR may have in preventing SIDS as a reason to take a CPR class.

Conclusion

You may discover that skimming, scanning, and marking text are skills that seem to occupy time. They do take some time to master, yet they will "pay off" for you in higher Verbal Reasoning scores. You will get faster at the techniques introduced in this chapter the more you practice them. Skimming, scanning, and marking text will likely improve your comprehension and help you answer more questions correctly. Find your own combination of techniques that works best for you—there is no one technique that works for everyone all the time.

Remember that the MCAT is a test very heavily weighed in reading. The science sections of the MCAT contain scientific passages which are each 200–300 or more words in length. Strong reading will likely improve your total MCAT performance!

Answers to Scanning Drills

Directions:
Score 4 points for each correct answer. 100 points equals 100%.

Scanning Drill 1

1.	stare	gawk
2.	little	tiny
3.	dull	stupid
4.	cord	rope
5.	chance	fortune
6.	plea	appeal
7.	amble	walk
8.	wait	bide
9.	divide	part
10.	group	gang
11.	jump	leap
12.	enjoy	like
13.	fat	stout
14.	unique	original
15.	character	nature
16.	surplus	remaining
17.	correct	true
18.	value	worth
19.	evil	wicked
20.	energy	vigor
21.	mind	brain
22.	tan	beige
23.	bay	gulf
24.	room	chamber
25.	dispel	scatter

Scanning Drill 2

1.	rough	smooth
2.	dirty	clean
3.	finger	toe
4.	ceiling	floor
5.	casual	formal
6.	day	night
7.	alive	deceased
8.	happy	miserable
9.	silly	solemn
10.	wonderful	awful
11.	awake	sleeping
12.	dark	light

13.	little	huge
14.	icy	hot
15.	wealth	poverty
16.	dismal	cheerful
17.	sweet	sour
18.	laugh	cry
19.	cautious	careless
20.	go	stop
21.	stale	fresh
22.	lazy	energetic
23.	always	never
24.	end	beginning
25.	luminous	dull

Chapter 7

Qualifiers and Distractors

You have already learned the strategies of reading the question stems, reading the passage carefully, and marking important points and concepts. Analyzing the questions and knowing how to use the process of elimination also can improve your verbal reasoning skills. Understanding how MCAT Verbal Reasoning passages use qualifying words and distractors will help you answer questions effectively and use the process of elimination successfully.

Qualifiers

Qualifiers are words that give the question stems or answer choices limited meaning. Success in verbal reasoning requires that you identify qualifiers in questions **before** evaluating possible answer choices. Try to identify words that narrow the scope or limit possible answer choices.

Question stems are designed to make only one of the four choices indisputably correct. Thus, the author of the question uses careful wording to limit the possible answers. When you can identify and understand qualifying words, you will be able to eliminate possible answers more easily and choose the best answer.

Although the temptation may be to hurry through the question stems to get to the four answer choices, there is an advantage to slowing down and thinking about the question phrase before moving to the answer choices. Make a habit of asking yourself the following two questions:

1. Is there a qualifying word that limits the possible answers? Look for words that indicate **positive absolutes, negative absolutes,** or **exceptions** (Table 7-1).

Table 7-1. Qualifying Words

Positive absolutes	Negative absolutes	Exceptions
All	None	Sometimes
Always	Never	At times
Best	Least	Most likely Frequently Seldom

2. Keeping the qualifying words in mind, can you come up with an answer, direction, or idea that addresses the question phrase **before** looking at the answer choices?

The advantage of this strategy is that you may have already formulated the correct answer in your mind and need only find it among the four choices. Also, if you have misread the stem, the choices given as answers will not make sense to you. If this happens, go back and examine the wording of the stem more carefully.

The **most common qualifiers** used on the Verbal Reasoning test are words that allow for **exceptions.** These qualifiers acknowledge a middle ground that does not reach either extreme. Because such terms stop short of absolutes, they more often denote a reasonable stance.

Five Strategic Points

The following five strategic points about qualifiers are important to keep in mind.

1. **Absolutes** such as *none, all, never,* and *always* often indicate an **incorrect** choice on the Verbal Reasoning test.
2. Qualifying words that allow room for **exceptions** are likely to signal a **correct** response. In addition to the exception words in Table 7-1, the following words also are imprecise enough to make statements difficult to contest and, therefore, likely to be correct: *few, often, some, probably, may, perhaps, might, generally, relative.*

   Similarly, phrases that indicate **qualification** may signal a **correct** response. A statement containing the following words or phrases is likely to be a correct answer: *among, seems to, would most likely, might suggest, might the author say.*
3. Stems that contain **exception phrases** such as *which of the following is NOT, which is LEAST supported,* or *all of the following EXCEPT* can be misread, even though the test maker often puts the exception word in **boldface,** *italics,* or CAPITAL letters. In fact, research shows that putting a word in a different typography actually makes some readers skip it. Do not allow yourself to skip these important words.
4. **Double negatives** in the stem also can be missed when the reader is hurried. Constructions such as *not unlike, not unimaginable,* and *cannot be dissociated* should be regarded like any double negative—as a positive.
5. **Abstract nouns** such as *theme, issue,* or *concern* and **abstract verbs** such as *reflected in* should be looked at carefully. Such generalizations do not imply that the passage is arguing for or against the idea, but simply that the idea appears as a concept within the passage.

Distractors

Distractors are incorrect answer choices (see Chapter 2). Distractors are frequently confusing or misleading because they are carefully constructed to simulate correct answers. Keep in mind that they are **not** randomly constructed by test writers. There are strategies for identifying common distractors used on the Verbal Reasoning test, and the important types of distractors are presented in this chapter.

On the Verbal Reasoning test, possibly only one of the four answers will be easily discarded. Sometimes, all four of the answer choices appear reasonable. To help you understand what helps test makers develop distractors, it is useful to categorize what tends to be incorrect about wrong answers. Look over the following common distractor types. When you begin practicing Verbal Reasoning passages, look for these common distractors and eliminate them as possible answer choices. This will help increase your Verbal Reasoning score!

Common Distractors

1. Sometimes test writers **repeat** or **restate** information from the passage in an answer choice **without answering the question** being asked. These choices are attractive because information is being drawn from the passage. Remember, if the choice does not answer the question, it is wrong.
2. The answer choice may be **too strong, overstating the idea** in the passage. Because the choice sounds partially correct and you are under a great time pressure, this type of answer choice can be compelling. Always ask yourself if the answer choice is overstated. Words that signal overstatement include: *all, must, most, only, always, most important, never, every, none, everywhere.*
3. Some answers use **words from the passage,** particularly terms that may be **unfamiliar** to you. These choices often reverse or imply a cause–effect relationship that is not supported by the passage.

The answer can misstate an idea in such a way that, although words from the passage appear in the answer choice, these words are not related to each other as they are in the passage.

4. An answer can make a **claim that is reasonably stated** and, although it does not answer the question, this choice is attractive to a hurried test taker. Such distractors tend to be generalizations with which no one could disagree but that do not answer the question.
5. Beware of the distractor that is either **pro** or **con** toward an argument and **represents only one side of the issue.** This choice might not support the author's overall viewpoint. The attraction to this choice is that the distractor actually appears in the passage and sounds true.
6. When **two distractors are almost synonymous,** they are both probably **incorrect.** Distractors with similar meanings often are used in inference questions regarding tone or purpose, where no single sentence supplies the answer. Your strategy should be to eliminate both synonymous choices, and focus on the remaining two choices. To use this strategy, **you must be certain that the two choices are indeed synonymous.** On the MCAT, you frequently will see two choices that are similar to each other but not synonymous. Two similar choices may be included in answers to see if you can determine gradations of meaning or connotation. In these cases, one of the choices is more accurate and is often the correct answer.
7. Distractors may use a word formed from a **key word** in the passage. The **root** of the key word may appear in a position of importance in the passage—at the end of the introduction, in a topic sentence, in the thesis—or it may be repeated in the passage. This makes it appear a likely choice as an answer.

Look at some examples of these distractors based on a passage that you have already read. Several questions follow the passage. Distractors will be identified and discussed.

Distractor Passage Exercise

The United States school system is in crisis. As middle-class families continue to move out of the city into the suburbs, the gap between the education of the rich and the poor continues to grow wider. Wealthy families have always had more options available to them than poor families have. Whereas a lack of financial resources leaves children of poor families trapped in inner-city schools, money has allowed the children of wealthy families to enroll in private schools, or to live in expensive houses in "good" public school districts.

"What is to be done" about the current state of the public school system has been a topic of debate for more than 50 years. Recently, failure to compete in international technological markets and an upcoming Presidential election have heightened the intensity of this debate. Conservatives have proposed a new plan called "Choice" that would operate on the model of the free market.

As the system now stands, the number of students per public school, largely determined by city districts, dictates the allocation of government funds in public schools. Choice would turn the United States school system into a mix of public, private, and parochial schools competing with one another for students and for government funding. By supplementing student tuition at private institutions, Choice would open private schools to more students. Advocates claim that public schools could then begin to compete with private schools for students. In turn, this competition would force public schools to increase their academic excellence in order to attract students with several schooling options open to them.

Proponents of Choice claim that competition for students, "customers," and government funding would insure excellence in schools. Families would be given vouchers to spend at the school, public or private, of their choice. Those in favor of Choice argue that the voucher system would allow families with meager funds to send their children to first-rate private institutions. They also claim that the program would give parents more options in selecting public schools for their children. In most states today, parents must send their children to the public school designated by their housing district. Under the proposed plan, parents would be free to choose the school they would like their children to attend.

Critics of Choice claim that the plan is mostly political rhetoric. Because private schools today are almost entirely full, the Choice plan would necessitate rapid and extensive rebuilding, something the government is not offering to fund. More radical critics of the plan claim that Choice would only make the education of the rich better, and the education of the poor worse. They claim that the government will not be able to provide the enormous funds necessary to make private education a real option for all families. Further, with government money all tied up in vouchers that will be inadequate for most, funds will not be available to help inner-city schools rebuild their programs. In a free market educational system, inner-city schools will never be competitive.

Before a truly "free" market can be opened, public school systems need to be restructured and refinanced. Before spending money on voucher experiments, the government needs to spend money on restructuring public schools.

Distractor Exercises: Part I

Directions:
The following questions are based on the passage. For each question, carefully review the answer choices, and see if you agree with the identification and analysis of the distractors. A brief discussion of each choice is given. In addition, each distractor is numbered type 1–7, based on the common distractor list given earlier in this chapter. Refer to the common distractor list to make sure that you agree with the identification of the distractor type.

1. The thesis being argued in this passage is that:

A. Choice would operate on the model of the free market system.
(*Discussion: Although this is true, it does not answer the question of thesis identification. This is distractor type 1.*)

B. most poor children in the United States receive an inferior education.
(*Discussion: This choice overstates the author's position. This is distractor type 2.*)

C. restructuring the public school system should be tried before vouchers.
(*Discussion: Best answer.*)

D. students in the United States public school system deserve the best education money can buy, regardless of how that is accomplished.
(*Discussion: Few could argue with the idealism of this statement, but it is too broad a generalization and does not define the central point of the argument. This is distractor type 4.*)

2. According to the passage, which of the following statements is true of vouchers?

A. They are inadequate for most families.
(Discussion: This view comes from critics of the plan and does not reflect the whole passage. This is distractor type 5.)

B. They are experimental.
(Discussion: Best answer.)

C. They will require the restructuring and refinancing of schools.
(Discussion: This reversal implies a causal relationship between vouchers and the author's own suggestions. This idea is not stated in the passage. This is distractor type 3.)

D. They will allow families to send their children to first-rate schools.
(Discussion: This view comes from proponents of Choice and does not reflect the whole passage or the author's view. This is distractor type 5.)

3. Based on the passage, which of the following statements would be most supported by proponents of Choice?

A. Requiring inner-city children to attend public schools
(Discussion: Note the use of the negative absolute word "requiring." This qualifying word helps identify this choice as a distractor. The passage emphasizes free choice. This is distractor type 2.)

B. Supporting an open discussion of legislation requiring that all low-income families be excluded from voucher programs
[Discussion: Note that the first part of this statement uses words that are soft in tone (i.e., open discussion) and later uses terms that are harsh and not supported by the passage (i.e., requiring, excluded). This choice misstates ideas from the passage. This is distractor type 3.]

C. Encouraging only government agencies to build more public schools
(Discussion: This statement uses the word "only," yet the passage emphasizes that proponents of Choice want more free enterprise to compete with the public sector. This answer choice uses words that are too strong and misstate the ideas given in the passage. This is distractor type 3.)

D. Encouraging more competition between the public and private school sectors
(Discussion: Best answer.)

4. Which term best describes the tone of the passage?

A. Quarrelsome
(Discussion: This choice can be eliminated in two ways. First, "quarrelsome" implies a negative tone. The passage is not negative. Second, this choice is synonymous with choice D. Remember that two synonymous choices are usually both incorrect. This is distractor type 6.)

B. Intense
(Discussion: Though the word "intensity" is used at the end of paragraph two, the passage itself sounds too reasoned to be termed intense. This is distractor type 7.)

C. Informed
(Discussion: Best answer.)

D. Combative
(Discussion: This choice can be eliminated in the same two ways that choice A was eliminated. This choice is synonymous with choice A. This is distractor type 6.)

Note: Correct answers to **tone questions** are typically not politically incorrect, sarcastic, strongly emotional, or derogatory. It is unlikely that unpopular, unethical, or extremely negative statements will be correct. A moderate tone, making a claim that seems to grow out of the entire passage, is more likely to be correct. In matters of tone, listen to the author's voice at the beginning and end of the passage. Notice adjectives—how does the writer characterize people, events, behaviors, and ideas? What sound emerges from all these adjectives used together? Keep in mind that tone means the attitude of the author toward the topic and, therefore, can include any description of emotion (e.g., reflective, clinical, conversational, regretful, celebratory, dismissive). If the tone is difficult to pinpoint, check topic sentences as well as the beginning and end of the passage. As always, when it comes down to one of two answers, treat each as a true/false choice. Look for flaws in both, and eliminate the lesser of the choices.

Distractor Exercises: Part II

The most effective way to understand the thinking involved in constructing distractors is to create some yourself. Reread the passage "Choice"; then write your own distractors from the following stems.

Directions:
In each of the questions, a question stem and the correct answer are provided. Create three distractor choices, and write them in the blanks. This exercise mimics the way the test writers create incorrect choices. Be sure to choose several different types of distractors, based on the common distractor list.

1. The word that best describes the author's attitude toward vouchers is:

A. skeptical.

B. ______________________________

C. ______________________________

D. ______________________________

Possible distractors: supportive, approving, encouraging, sympathetic, understanding, reassuring, obstinate, biased, unyielding, bigoted, assertive, opinionated.

2. According to the passage, causes of the educational gap in the United States include:

A. financial disparity between families.

B. ______________________________

C. ______________________________

D. ______________________________

Possible distractors:
intelligence levels among children.
scholastic excellence in inner-city schools.
more opportunities for children of poor families.
fewer opportunities for children of wealthy families.
a crisis for the United States school system.
expensive houses have "good" school districts.
poor families have a lack of financial resources.

3. According to the passage, the voucher system most resembles the "free market" in that:

A. competition would increase the overall quality of services.

B. ______________________________

C. ______________________________

D. ______________________________

Possible distractors:
Private schools would be open to more students.
Supplementation of student tuition at private schools would increase enrollments in the private sector.
The United States school system would become mixed.
There would be less competition among private schools.
Competition would decrease public school enrollments.
All students would compete for private school entrance.

Chapter 8

Eye and Hand Movements for Faster, More Effective Reading

Introduction

The eye and hand movements introduced in this chapter are advocated by speed-reading courses, and most students find great value in some of these techniques. Work through this chapter carefully. After practicing some of the techniques taught here, decide on which of the methods improves your speed. These techniques can be useful, but they are **optional.**

In order to read rapidly, our eyes must move quickly over printed material, without moving back over material we have already read. However, most of us are in the habit of reading words, sentences, whole paragraphs, and pages over again because we feel we have missed some information. Sometimes we read sections of a reading passage over a second time because we have been taught that in order to fully comprehend a text, we need to read every single word and understand everything perfectly as we read. These **regressions increase the time** spent reading and may **detract** from our concentration. Instead of keeping our attention on what is coming next in a text and on overall comprehension, we waste time repeating our reading.

On the MCAT, the more words you have to read in a passage, the more time it takes. Increasing your reading speed on the Verbal Reasoning test requires that you read fewer individual words and more segments or phrases of words (word blocks). This chapter gives you some new strategies to read words in word blocks. You will also be encouraged to use your peripheral vision to increase the span of your reading without moving your eyes over the entire line of text. Finally, you will be presented with five powerful hand movement techniques to increase your reading speed.

Your goal on the Verbal Reasoning section of the MCAT is to read as **fast** as you can and with as **much comprehension as possible.** When you read through each Verbal Reasoning passage the first time, always keep your eyes moving ahead, toward the end of the text. This will not be easy at first because over the years, you probably have learned to move your eyes slowly over a text, moving backwards frequently. Breaking old reading habits takes practice. In this chapter, you will work on practicing faster, more efficient eye movements and using hand movements to increase eye movement speed.

When practicing more efficient eye movements, you might use your eyes alone, or you might use your hand to guide your eyes along. First, begin with practicing eye movements alone; then work on incorporating hand movements. As you learn these methods, you will discover which is best for you, but be sure to try all of the methods.

Eye Movements

Your eyes move in short, sudden movements across the page. Each time your eye moves, it takes in a group of words, and the more words you can read in each eye movement, the faster you will read. Also, when you practice taking in more words at once, your comprehension improves because you are reading words in association with other words.

Look at the difference between the number of words the following types of readers see at a given interval. Each reader in these examples reads from one mark (/) to the next. Move your eyes from one mark to the next to get a sense of how fast each reader is reading.

Word-by-Word

In / November / the / leaves / have / completely / fallen / off / the / trees / and / the / grass / is / dormant / and / gray, / making / the / world / look / like / it / is / preparing / for / a / long / sleep.

A Little Faster

A combination / of the / increase of / the population / over the / years (from / 193 million / in 1965 / to 260 / million by / 1995) and / an increase / in our / production of / garbage that / make up / the United States' / enormous stockpile / of solid waste.

Faster Yet

The colonized live / in the constantly / ambiguous state of / the oppressed, and / some attempt to / escape it by / becoming members of / authority, like police / officers; however, Memmi / states that escape / from oppression for / the colonized is / ultimately impossible.

Speed-Reader

Isak Dinesen, / Baroness Karen von Blixen-Finecke, / was an eccentric, influential woman / who, because of the many / colorful facets of her personality, / affected the lives of all / who knew her or / came in contact with her work.

To become a faster reader, you need to train yourself to read **three to five words (a phrase)** in a **single eye span.** Now look at an exercise that might help you to read in phrases. In this exercise, a section of an MCAT passage has been broken up into phrases, and these phrases have been lined up vertically in columns. Try reading each phrase as fast as you can. Remember, try to take in the whole line at once.

Single Eye-Span Exercise 1

How to ride a bicycle
successfully is much more
complicated than most riders
believe. Professional bicycle racers
know several tricks of the
trade. First and foremost, there
is the issue of safety. Helmets
are mandatory. Currently, fewer than
15% of all bicyclists wear helmets.
(Fewer than 5% of all children do!)
That statistic is especially sad
considering that over 90% of all fatal
bicycle accidents are from head injuries
and most could have been
prevented had only the rider
worn a helmet. Nowadays helmets
are made of such lightweight

materials that overheating because
your head is covered should no
longer be a hazard.

Reading phrases of three to five words, instead of each individual word increases your reading time. Keep this kind of phrase reading in mind as you read more of this passage in regular paragraph form. Remember, make your eyes see whole phrases. Read as quickly as you can!

Single Eye-Span Exercise 2

Some professional bicyclists so / want to decrease the amount / of extra weight they carry that / they remove all the reflectors / on their bicycles. Of course, / one should never do this. / It is always important to / be easily visible to passersby. / You should have reflectors on both / the front and rear tires, as well as / on the back of the bicycle. / Most bicycle shoes also have / reflective material sewn on. / Having a headlight and perhaps / a taillight too, is another good idea / because you never know when / you might be out bicycling / at nightfall or during a storm. / And if the light's power is generated / by the bicycle, then you / never have to worry about batteries / going dead just when / you need the light.

Newspapers and magazines are good for practicing eye-span reading because they have the narrow column format that is conducive to this kind of speed-reading practice. Make a conscious effort to read several articles from a newspaper each day, timing yourself and making yourself read more words in each eye span.

Also, you can practice speed reading using Columbia Review study materials. Three full-length practice tests are included in this book. Three more full-length tests are found in the *Columbia Review Intensive MCAT Preparation* book. The Columbia Review Home Study Course provides many additional Verbal Reasoning tests for practice. Remember that practice is always the best way to prepare for the Verbal Reasoning section of the MCAT. When you are taking a practice MCAT or the actual test, try using eye span when you first look at each paragraph of the passage to gain a quick understanding of the paragraphs.

Hand Movements

Why use your hands to increase your reading speed? Although there is some controversy about eye–hand reading, if properly used, it can be one of the fastest ways to increase your reading speed. There are **four top reasons** to use hand movements:

1. Running your hand down a page of reading material automatically leads your eyes down the type. It prevents you from slowing down or pausing.
2. The hand movements control your reading speed.
3. Moving your hand across a page helps you focus on important key words and ideas, while ignoring unimportant details.
4. Hand movements help many readers stay focused and improve concentration.

Using your **hand as a pacer** to guide your eyes can **increase your reading speed.** Hand movements are effective at increasing reading speed because your eyes have something to follow, and you can easily control how fast your hand is moving. Following your hand as you read is not easy to do at first, but with practice (and if it suits your reading style), using your hand as a pacer can feel natural. Now, look at some specific methods for hand movements.

Conventionalism suggests that law is never complete. There are always new circumstances

presenting new challenges which have never been considered, much less settled, by

conventional legislative bodies. This incompleteness means that judges must decide some

cases as best they can, but without relying on conventionally approved legislative outcomes.

Figure 8–1. The straight single-line method.

Introductory Methods

Method 1: Straight Single-Line Method

This is the **most common method** used by speed readers because it is simple to use. It is not as fast as some of the other methods presented in this chapter, but it requires less practice to master. In this method, the hand is moved from left to right under each line. You can choose either the index finger or the middle finger as the lead pointer. The eyes should be focused just to the right of the finger. At the end of a line, the hand is moved to the beginning of the next line without lifting the hand much from the page. Repeat the process, moving the hand down the page. Concentrate on keeping your elbow close to your body and your head still. The single-line method is illustrated in Figure 8-1.

Try reading the following paragraph from a practice MCAT while moving your hand from left to right under each line as you try to read. Use your **hand** in a **relaxed position, gliding your fingertips** across the page as quickly as you can.

> A bicycle should fit you properly. To determine whether the bicycle is the correct height, stand next to the bicycle. The crossbar should be the same height as the top of the inseam of your pants. To determine whether the bicycle is the proper length, you should sit on the seat with your hands on the handlebars, and glance down with your head facing forward. The handlebars should block your view of the front tire sprocket. Finally, the seat should be adjusted such that your heels just barely graze each pedal when it is in its lowest position when your legs are fully extended.

It probably felt awkward to use your hand. You may have found yourself looking at your hand more than at the text, but with practice you will become accustomed to seeing your hand. Try not to move your head as you read from left to right; keep your eyes on the line of text.

Comprehension will improve as you practice this new technique, but at first you may feel you cannot remember much of what you read. This probably is the result of being distracted by your hand. But by moving your hand quickly over the lines of the text, you are actually training your eyes to move more quickly. Comprehension will come as you learn to read and retain what you read at a faster rate.

Method 2: Gentle Curve Single-Line Method

There is a simple modification of the single-line method that some students prefer. It is called the gentle curve single-line method. In this technique, the pointer finger is gently curved from the end of the line to the beginning of the next line without lifting the pointer finger from the page (Figure 8-2). The curves are

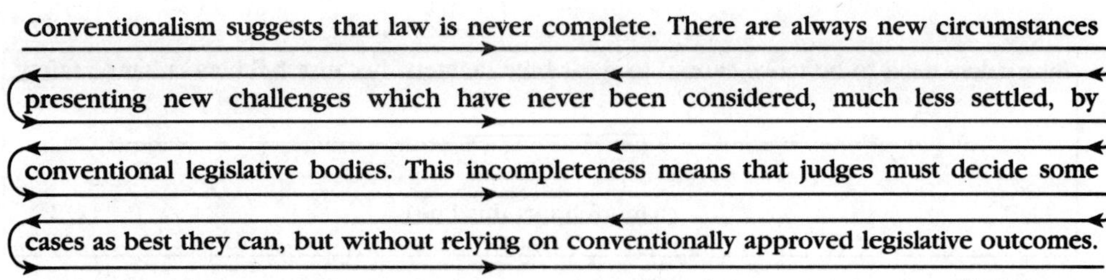

Figure 8–2. The gentle curve single-line method.

sweeping and fluid in motion. As with the straight method, the eyes should stay focused to the right of the pointer finger.

Now try applying this second method to a reading passage from a Verbal Reasoning test. Remember to use a gentle curve motion to move from the end of one line to the beginning of the next line.

> Arising from nothing, human thought takes an incredible leap. From the abstract comes the concrete, and that which was never possible before is suddenly before our eyes. From the void of nothingness comes with shocking tangibility the real. This is the essence of mankind's power over his environment. He can place himself in an alternate existence where all is possible. From the enigma of complex neurochemical reactions comes thought—but thought cannot be adequately explained with balanced equations and chemical interactions. From whence does this ability arise? How do we reconcile our physical existence with our metaphysical one?

As you practice, you may find that the loops your finger makes are becoming bigger and more fluid. There are several hand movements variations that may help you to read more material in less time. None of these patterns work unless you practice, and you should try each one to determine with which you are the most comfortable.

Power-Reading Strategies to Use with Hand Movements

You can use your peripheral vision strategically when using hand movements. Most readers can easily see at least three words to the left or right from where their eye is focused. When you use your hand to guide your eyes, start by placing your hand ½ inch to the right of the left margin. As your hand sweeps to the right, end your hand movement ½ inch to the left of the right margin. This will save you time without decreasing your comprehension.

1. Start reading about two to three words into the line of type, about ½ inch from the left margin.
2. Stop reading two or three words before the end of the line of type, about ½ inch from the right margin.

Read the line in Figure 8-3, but start your hand and eyes ½ inch from the beginning of the line of print and ½ inch before the end of the line.

Bike riders need to be more careful to wear bike helmets, because helmets enhance safety.

(1/2″) **(hand follows this line)** **(1/2″)**

Figure 8–3. Power-reading strategy.

When you look at a letter or a word, your eyes actually see all the area surrounding it—using your peripheral vision, you can read several words at a time. Look at the word "need" in this line. Along with it, you can read "Bike riders." The same goes for "helmets"—you can read "enhance safety" at the end of the line.

Try reading the following passage. Starting ½ inch in, use your hand under each line, ending each line ½ inch from the end of the print. Keep your head still, and move your eyes and hand only. Remember to move your hand as quickly as possible.

What equipment should you take along when riding? A quart or more of water is needed if your trip is longer than a few miles. This can ride in a cage attached to your frame. A patch kit for fixing flat tires is also useful. It should contain three "spoons" for getting the tire off the frame, a small piece of sandpaper for filing down the ridges on the inner tube so that the patch can form a tight seal, several different size patches, and some epoxy glue. The patch kit can fit neatly into a small carrying case tied to the base of your seat. Of course, no patch kit is complete without an air pump to inflate the fixed tire. You should only use these portable air pumps for blowing up tires on the road because most tires require 90 pounds per square inch pressure, which is extremely difficult to manage if you are pushing air in using your arms alone. Underinflated tires will not only slow you down, but also could cause damage to the rims of your bicycle.

Get into the habit of hand movements by practicing on magazine or newspaper articles. You also can practice these techniques in the practice tests included in this book.

Advanced Techniques

These techniques are more complicated than the earlier two methods. However, they are often more powerful. Some students find that with practice, these hand techniques are great tools for increasing reading speed.

Method 3: Center Method

This is a useful technique because it takes full advantage of your field of vision. It allows you to read fewer words because you read in blocks and is one of the fastest techniques. The method is relatively simple. Place your pointer finger on the center of the printed page and focus your eyes in front of your finger. Move your finger from left to right as you move your eyes. When your finger reaches an inch or so from the right margin, swing it to the middle of the next line. This technique is great for use on the MCAT Verbal Reasoning section because the reading passages are in a two-column format. The lines are fairly short, with an average of about 10 words per line. By focusing on the center of each line and using the center method, you can read rapidly by seeing words in blocks. A schematic for this technique is shown in Figure 8-4.

Now try the center method on a paragraph from a Verbal Reasoning test.

> It is an excellent solution to the security dilemma in part due to its inherently stable nature. It is built on a system whereby all members of the organization rely on all other members of the organization to come to their aid in a time of trouble. The stability arises from the desire of all the actors to maintain the peace through nonaggression. Because every state in the world ascribes to the same goal, the peace is ensured. If, for example, a power were to attempt to tip the scales in its favor, the other nations would correct the imbalance and ensure continued security. Besides providing a stable alternative to the security dilemma, it is also an excellent deterrent to aggression. When trying to reduce the likelihood of war, it is essential to reduce the incentive for conflict to the lowest possible levels. Collective security deters any state from attacking another by ensuring swift and devastating retribution for acts of aggression by other members. War is a product of conflict, and so eliminating potential conflict eliminates a precursor to war.

Method 4: Right-Angle Method

This is an advanced technique that works for some readers. It is somewhat more complex than the earlier techniques, but with practice, this method can be effective. Starting at the left side of the print, go under the line with the index finger only, moving to the right. At the end of the line, lift the finger and place it directly above about two lines up on the page (at right). Move the finger downward on a slant, going toward the left to finish six lines down, at the beginning of the line (at left). Lift the finger and place it directly above about two lines up on the page at the beginning of the line (at left). Move the finger straight across

Start Here

Conventionalism suggests that law is never complete. There are always new circumstances

presenting new challenges which have never been considered, much less settled, by

conventional legislative bodies. This incompleteness means that judges must decide some

cases as best they can, but without relying on conventionally approved legislative outcomes.

The results of this type of legislative action is yet to be evaluated impartially.

Figure 8–4. The center method.

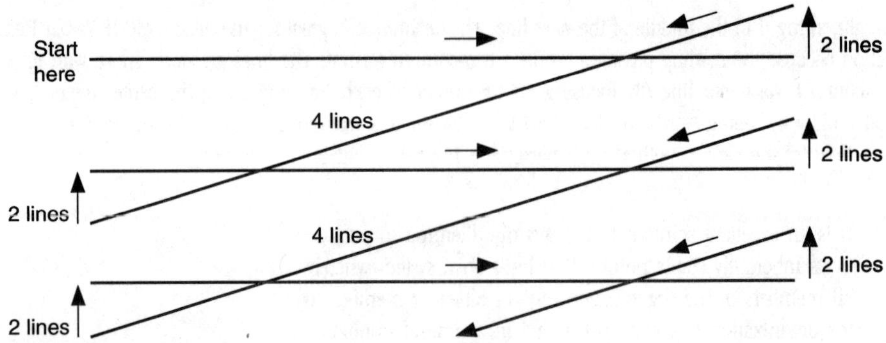

Figure 8–5. The right-angle method.

to the right under the line. Continue and repeat entire hand movement (Figure 8-5). Practice this hand movement for a few seconds.

Try the right-angle method on a paragraph from a Verbal Reasoning test.

The year 1815 had marked the end of a period of American development. Up to this time, the life of the continent had been molded largely by forces from Europe; but with the conclusion of the War of 1812 against England, America turned in upon herself and with her back to the Atlantic, looked toward the West. The years following the Peace of Ghent are full of the din of the Westward advance. In politics, the vehement struggles of Federalist and Republican were replaced by what a contemporary journalist called "the era of good feelings." But underneath the calm surface of the first decade lay the bitter rivalry of sectional interests that were soon to assume permanent and organized party forms. As in all postwar periods, the major political issue was that of finance. The ideas of Alexander Hamilton on protection and banking were reluctantly accepted by the Republican administration under the stress of war conditions.

Method 5: Curved-Angle Method

This technique is a modification of the right-angle method. The hand movement is done exactly like the right-angle method except that the index finger remains on the page. Do not lift the finger to place it two lines above. Instead, curve it around upward so that loops are made around the beginnings and the ends of the lines that take place in about two lines (Figure 8-6). Practice for a few seconds.

Now try the curved-angle method on a paragraph from a Verbal Reasoning test.

Mankind's ability to function in the abstract is his greatest triumph. To merely *conceive* is an incredible feat. It requires an incredible array of faculties that have never been even closely replicated. Indeed, the capacities of the human brain are only superficially understood. Without a working knowledge about the inception of thought, we continue to utilize it frequently and easily. We are the sole proprietor of our thought, and yet we have no owner's manual or instruction book on how to use it, or what makes it tick. We simply *do* it. The process is a mystery, but the ability is undeniably real. Thoughts that are without boundary are somehow contained in the physical parameters of our brain.

These last two hand movements (right-angle and curved-angle methods) direct your eyes in a specific pattern. They are used best whenever you want to emphasize a particular line, such as in previewing or reading informational material.

To use any of these hand movements, you will need to practice as much as you can to become comfortable; with comfort will come greater speed and comprehension. As you read a text, vary hand movements you use to keep yourself attentive to your reading task.

If you need to keep yourself physically active as you read—for example, if you find you need to fiddle with a pencil or bounce your leg as you read—these hand movements might work very well for you. You can improve your reading speed and comprehension by substituting hand movements for the other movements. If you do not use hand movements already, they may not come naturally. Hand movements will feel more natural with practice. See if they work well for you!

Here is another MCAT practice passage for you to read. Time yourself as you read, and try using one of the new techniques from this chapter. Be sure to use eye-span techniques (read words in blocks), and try one of the hand techniques. Push yourself to read **fast** for your best time yet. Do not concentrate on individual words—look at phrases and whole paragraphs.

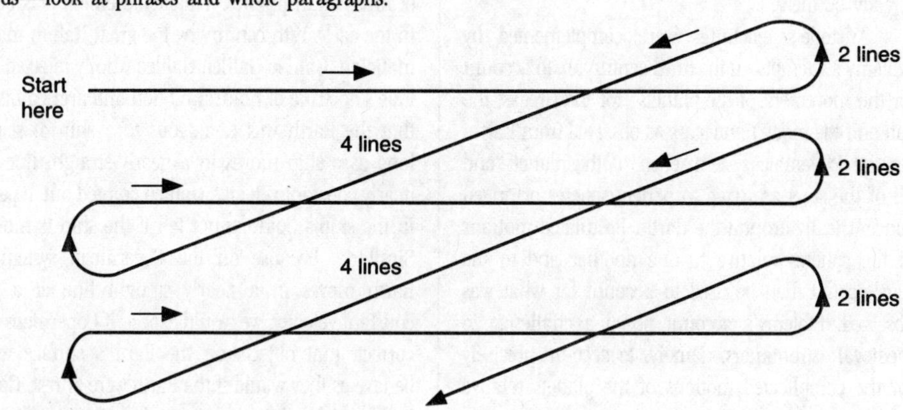

Figure 8–6. The curved-angle method.

Directions:
Record the times that you start and finish reading this passage in minutes and seconds. Subtract your starting time from your finishing time to find your total.

MCAT Practice Passage VI

	Minutes	Seconds
Your finishing time:		
Your starting time:		(subtract)
Your total time:		

Record your starting time now, and begin reading.

MCAT Practice Passage VII

In the 16th and 17th centuries, the universe changed dramatically. The geocentric and geostatic worldview of the 15th century was replaced with one that described the Earth as hurling around a fixed sun at a high speed. This revolutionary change is one of the most fascinating and important episodes in the history of science.

European intellectuals inherited a worldview derived from Aristotle, the great philosopher of ancient Athens. Aristotle held that the Earth was composed primarily of two elements, earth and water, and that the natural motion of these elements was rectilinear and toward the center of the universe; for if it were not at the center, it would be moving there. But because it is obviously not moving, it must already be there.

Aristotle's teachings were complemented by Ptolemy's attempts, in the third century AD, to account for the movement of the planets (for the Greeks, the sun and the moon) and stars as observed from Earth. On the Ptolemaic system, each of the planets and all of the stars are fixed to perfect spheres arranged concentrically around the Earth. Postulated motions of the spheres relative to one another and to the Earth could then be used to account for what was observed. Ptolemy's account posed a challenge to medieval astronomers, namely, to account precisely for the complicated motions of the planets relative to the stars.

This "saving of the appearances" proved difficult indeed. As explanatory attempts grew increasingly complex and ad hoc, King Alphonso X reportedly commented, in the 13th century, that if the Lord Almighty had consulted him, he "would have recommended something simpler."

Alphonso's sentiment was shared by Nicholas Copernicus, a Polish canon. Copernicus experimented with the Ptolemaic system by exchanging the position of the sun and the Earth. This simple alteration reaped immediate advantages. Things that were difficult to explain on the Ptolemaic system, such as the fact that Venus and Mars always appeared near the sun or that some planets occasionally displayed a backward or "retrograde" motion against the fixed stars, simply "fell out" of the Copernican system. In 1543, the last year of his life, Copernicus published his system in a work titled, *On the Revolutions of the Heavenly Spheres.*

Although impressed by its advantages, astronomers tended to accept Copernicus' system only as a calculating device. How, they asked, could the Earth really move? Wouldn't everything fly off? Acceptance of the Copernican system awaited the reformulation of Artisotelian physics. This achievement was begun in the early 17th century by the great Italian mathematician, Galileo Galilei. Galileo wholly rejected Aristotle's doctrine of natural motion and argued instead that the Earth was analogous to a ship at sea. So long as a ship moves in a nearly straight line at a nearly constant velocity, Galileo pointed out, a person in the ship's hold cannot tell if the ship is moving. Similarly, because on the Copernican system the Earth moves in a nearly straight line at a near constant velocity, we would expect, if Copernicus were correct, that objects on the Earth's surface would behave as they would if the Earth were at rest. Galileo had formulated a precursor to the principle of inertia.

Acceptance of the Copernican system followed rapidly on the elaboration of Galileo's physics. Some 50 years after Galileo, a young Isaac Newton would formulate the new physics with unprecedented rigor, and in the process lay to rest any remaining objections to the Earth's motion. No reasonable person thereafter could hold that our Earth was at rest at the center of the universe; indeed, after Copernicus, Galileo, and Newton, the world would never be the same.

Word Count: 589

Directions:
Record the time you finished reading in the space provided at the beginning of the passage. Subtract your starting time from your finishing time to find out how long it took you to read it.

Your reading rate is: ______________________.

Comprehension Questions

1. According to the passage, a major problem faced by medieval astronomers was to:

A. explain how it could be that the Earth moved.
B. show how the Copernican model of the universe explained the apparent motions of the planets.
C. show how the Ptolemaic model of the universe "saved the appearances."
D. predict the location of the sun and moon as they appeared from Earth.

2. Based on the information in the passage, which of the following statements, if true, would provide evidence against the Copernican system?

A. The motion of Mars, Venus, and the moon cannot be accounted for on the Copernican system.
B. Most people in the holds of real ships can tell if and how the ship they are in is moving.
C. The Copernican system is significantly simpler than its competitors.
D. Sixty years after its formulation, only a handful of people accepted the Copernican system.

3. A good title for this passage would be:

A. "The Newtonian Achievement."
B. "Galileo and the Principle of Inertia."
C. "Explanation in Astronomy."
D. "The Revolution in Astronomy."

4. Which of the following statements best summarizes the conclusion of the argument that the passage attributes to Galileo?

A. If the Earth were moving, objects on the surface of the Earth would not fly off.
B. If the Copernican system were true, objects on the surface of the Earth would not fall off.
C. The Earth is an inertial system.
D. The Earth moves.

5. Information in the passage suggests that:

A. Copernicus lived after Aristotle but before King Alfonso X.
B. Aristotle and Ptolemy were contemporaries.
C. Galileo lived before Newton and after Copernicus.
D. Newton and Galileo were contemporaries.

6. Which of the following does the passage cite as evidence for the truth of the Copernican system over the Ptolemaic?

I. The formulation of the new physics by Isaac Newton
II. The Ptolemaic system becoming very complicated
III. The Copernican system explaining the apparent proximity of Venus and Mars to the sun
IV. The Copernican system accounting more naturally for the retrograde motion of some planets

A. III only
B. II and IV only
C. I and III only
D. I, III, and IV only

7. The passage suggests that:

A. Galileo's system of physics led to the acceptance of the Copernican system.
B. the ability to account for retrograde motion led to the acceptance of the Copernican system.
C. the Copernican system was ultimately accepted because it was simpler.
D. the Copernican system accounted precisely for all known astronomical observations.

8. Which of the following statements best summarizes the conclusion of the argument that the passage attributes to Aristotle?

A. The Earth is not in motion.
B. The Ptolemaic system is probably true.
C. The Earth is at the center of the universe.
D. The Earth has a rectilinear natural motion.

Directions:
Correct your answers by using the Answers and Explanations section. Allow 12.5 percentage points for each correct answer.

MCAT Practice Passage VII Comprehension Score and Reading Rate

Your comprehension test score __________%. *Your reading rate* ______________.

Discussion of MCAT Practice Passage VII

Notice that this passage is expository; expect it to explain something to you. In passages of this type, make a mental map or simple notations in the margins outlining the flow of information. Notice that this passage is also organized chronologically. The first paragraph states that in the 16th and 17th centuries, there were revolutionary changes in views of the universe. This should tell you to expect more detail in the coming paragraphs about these changes. The second paragraph discusses Aristotle and his belief that the earth is moving toward the center of the universe. The next paragraph then discusses the fact that Ptolemy's beliefs complemented Aristotle's and accounted for the complicated motions of the planets relative to the stars. Paragraph four is brief and serves as a bridge to the next section of the passage by explaining that King Alphonso X wanted a simpler explanation than the ones that had been introduced so far. Paragraph five says that Copernicus altered Ptolemy's theory by switching the sun and the Earth, attempting to simplify the theory. The sixth paragraph discusses Galileo's theory that the Earth does not move and shows how this theory was born out of Aristotle's original idea. Then, paragraph seven leads to Newton's theory of physics and the final refutation that the Earth is at rest in the middle of the universe. This passage moves through time to show the evolution of views about the universe.

Answers and Explanations to MCAT Practice Passage VII

1. **C** According to the passage, medieval astronomers predated the Copernican system, and they did not think that the Earth moved. They wished to predict the location of the sun and moon, but they wanted to explain the locations of the other planets as well, all within the Ptolemaic system.
2. **A** Real ships move neither uniformly nor linearly, so they are what the passage describes as Galileo imagining. Nor does the passage suggest that being simple or not being accepted count against the truth of an astronomical theory. The passage does suggest that not accounting for the appearances of planets counts against an astronomical theory.
3. **D** The passage discusses Galileo and Newton only briefly and does not discuss explanation exactly. The first and last paragraphs suggest that the passage addresses a revolution in astronomy.
4. **B** According to the passage, Galileo did not argue that no matter how the Earth was moving, objects would not fall off it; nor did he argue that the Earth does in fact move. The passage does not attribute to Galileo any claim about inertial systems. Instead, it presents Galileo as arguing for a particular consequence of the Copernican system.
5. **C** The passage states that Copernicus died in 1543, well before the early 17th century when Galileo worked. It also states that Newton was young 50 years after Galileo.
6. **D** Retrograde motion and the ability to account for the positions of Venus and Mars are explicitly mentioned as advantages of the Copernican system over the Ptolemaic, and Newton's achievement is described as shutting the door on objections to Copernicanism. But the argument does not present complexity as a reason to consider one theory more likely to be true than another.
7. **A** The acceptance of the Copernican system is described as following readily on Galileo's physics; the suggestion is that the latter caused the former.
8. **C** That the Earth is not in motion and has a rectilinear motion are premises of Aristotle's argument, which concludes that the Earth is at the center of the universe. The passage also makes it clear that Aristotle predated the Ptolemaic system and, therefore, could not argue for its truth.

Remember, although hand movements may not be for everyone, they may work for you. Particularly if you have a heavy load of reading to do, hand movements may serve a double purpose: they may help you read faster, and they may help you stay alert and active. Being an active reader makes you a faster, more effective reader by keeping you involved in what you are reading.

Chapter 9

Speed-Reading Scientific and Other Specialized Material

One of the main differences between reading an article in a magazine and reading scientific material is that the magazine article uses language and vocabulary that a general audience can understand, whereas scientific material uses a language and vocabulary that is specialized. Scientific reading passages frequently are found on the MCAT, particularly in the Physical and Biological Sciences sections. These sections often are densely filled with facts, details, formulas, and examples. This specialized language is meant for a particular audience—premedical students. There are some great techniques to improve your reading of scientific and other technical MCAT passages. In this chapter, you will learn a method for making scientific and other difficult reading passages easier to comprehend.

Technique for Speed-Reading Scientific or Technical Material

Here is a good method to try when speed-reading scientific or technical material:

1. **Preview** the passage, skimming for the main ideas and structure. Take a few seconds to mark key places in the text. Note important topic sentences, key words, important phrases, and important concepts.
2. **Mark** any words that are unfamiliar to you and that seem to be important to the central topic of the passage. Remember to use a mark that is different from the marks you use for other details. Do not search hard for these specialized words, but let them jump out at you; then mark them.
3. After the preview and before good comprehension reading, go through the text to find the words you marked, and look at the sentence where you found them. You can usually **decipher the meaning of the word from the context** of the sentence.
4. Now you are ready to **read quickly** through the **entire passage** for good comprehension.

Try this technique when reading scientific passages on the MCAT. Also, try this approach as you practice reading MCAT Verbal Reasoning passages, particularly passages that seem to contain terms or words you do not know. Recognizing unfamiliar words right away and attempting to define them before reading the passage increases your speed because you do not need to stop as often when you do not recognize a word. Although you will not have a dictionary or glossary to look up these unfamiliar words, you can look at the sentence that contains the word, and make an inference about the word's general definition from the **context** of the sentence.

Of course, it is wise to brush up on your vocabulary before taking the MCAT. Although the vocabulary used on the Verbal Reasoning test is not too difficult for a native English reader with a college-level vocabulary, some students with a weakness in vocabulary find the words used in MCAT passages challenging. If your English vocabulary is a weakness, one way to build your vocabulary is to work through the MCAT Verbal

Reasoning Vocabulary Development Program in the appendix of this book. If you have the time before the MCAT, you can also increase your vocabulary and practice your speed and comprehension by reading as much as possible. Pick a book you are interested in that also seems to be written in a style that is slightly more difficult than what you usually read. Keeping a dictionary handy, read through the book as quickly as you can, previewing to find words that are new to you. Always look for new words, and get in the habit of writing them down, then looking them up in your dictionary. When you take practice MCATs, you will be more accustomed to new words, and your comprehension will increase as a result. Taking a bit of extra time to look up new words when you encounter them will save you time and effort later.

Skimming to Preview Content

Effective skimming is one of the most valuable speed-reading techniques for scientific or technical MCAT passages. When you skim, read groups of words or parts of sentences rather than individual words. Always look for key words, numbers, and graphics, if there are any. Think about the importance of the word groups and concepts. Thinking about the passage in advance of formally reading it gives you time to place meaning and significance on the passage. This ultimately helps your comprehension. When you skim technical passages, focus on these parts:

1. Title
2. Author
3. Headings
4. Footnotes or endnotes
5. Subheads
6. Works cited
7. Charts
8. Graphs
9. Drawings
10. Material that is indented, numbered, or set off from the rest of the text in any way

Make markings in the margin of the passage, underline, or circle important key words, phrases, and concepts. Use a marking system such that you know why you marked a particular section of the passage while skimming (see Chapter 6).

The following passage may contain words or terms that are unfamiliar. Be sure to first skim the passage marking key words, phrases, and concepts. Then mark any words that are not familiar. Use the context of the sentence to determine a likely meaning for these words. After these preliminary steps, read the passage for good comprehension and speed.

Technical Scientific Passage 1

The United States Department of Energy has awarded $9.2 million to a collaboration of scientists from Howard University, University of Michigan, and AT&T Bell Labs for research at the Advanced Photon Source (APS) of Argonne National Laboratory. The research grant is believed by many to represent the culmination of a long period of intense speculation, arbitration, and collaboration.

University of Michigan Physics Professor Roy Clarke, director of the Applied Physics Program, will co-direct this project with Howard University's Dr. Walter Lowe and Dr. Ronald Pindak of AT&T Bell Labs. The grant provides 4 years of research at the APS, a giant 7 GeV positron storage ring designed for the production of high-brilliance x-ray synchrotron radiation. Upon completion in

1998, the APS will be the world's brightest light source. The lumination provided by the project is expected to be disproportionate to the subdued expectations of speculators.

The accelerator, two-thirds of a mile in circumference, will allow researchers to carry out time-resolved studies and evaluations of materials under real dynamic conditions for the first time and makes it possible for them to investigate microscopic behavior of various physical and chemical processing, behavior or materials under stress and structural relaxation, the kinetic mechanisms of growth, and the real-time evolution of chemical reactions. The team will work with two fully instrumented beamlines, one involving a bend magnet source and the other an undulator, with high-resolution analyzers and fast array detectors used for time-resolved scattering. "Among the most intriguing aspects of synchrotron radiation from an undulator device," Professor Clarke explains, "are its laser-like qualities of extreme brightness and coherence." Several experiments will exploit these characteristics, including photon correlation spectroscopy and x-ray holographic imaging.

The researchers expect that their work will draw interest from many disciplines. As Dr. Lowe notes, "physicists, chemists, materials scientists, and engineers all have a different perspective on the dynamics of materials." And Clarke points out that students—graduate and undergraduate—will have good access to the research equipment as well, as high-speed communications will link the participating institutions to the APS facility.

Homer A. Neal, Vice President for Research at the University of Michigan, says, "We are delighted to participate with Howard University and AT&T Bell Labs in this cutting edge advanced materials research. This project stands as an example of outstanding interinstitutional collaboration. . . . The implications for both basic and applied research are excellent."

Adapted from E.T. Elliot, *Modern Physics News, Spring 1997.*

Directions:
Answer the following questions to see if you understood what you read.

1. What is the main idea of the article?

____

____

2. In your own words, how is the grant to be used?

____

____

3. What are some of the benefits of this grant?

____

____

Answers to Scientific Passage Exercise 1

1. From information given in the first paragraph, you should be able to write a sentence that gives the main idea of the article: The Department of Energy gives a grant to scientists from Howard, U-M, and AT&T for photon research at APS. Your summary does not necessarily need to include all the details because on a first read, you should mainly search for general ideas before you move into names, dates, and specifics.
2. The passage indicates that the grant provides 4 years of research at the APS, in which time-resolved studies and evaluations of materials will be conducted with an accelerator and positron storage ring.
3. What are some of the benefits of this grant? This question also can be answered in your own words in the form of a list. Four years of research will allow researchers to carry out many studies under certain conditions for the first time; the research will draw interest from many disciplines; students will have access to the research equipment. Put the list together something like this: The grant will provide funding such that researchers can perform novel studies for the first time. The grant will also allow teaching opportunities, valuable collaboration between scientists, and interinstitutional collaboration.

In reading any kind of technical material with which you are not familiar, try to explain the main points to yourself in your own words. Think, "In other words . . . " as if you were trying to explain the points to a classmate. Again, this explanation does not need to reproduce all the details from the original source, but it should give the gist of the reading in language that you understand best.

Here is another passage excerpt:

Technical Scientific Passage 2

Recent genetic studies have demonstrated that many craniosynostosis syndromes, including Crouzon's disease, Apert syndrome, Pfeiffer syndrome, and Jackson-Weiss syndrome, are linked to mutations of cellular receptors. It is believed that a family of cell-surface receptors mediates a complex series of functions in both embryonic development and growth. These functions include control of cellular proliferation, differentiation, cellular migration and survival. The FGF receptor 2, in particular, has been shown to be important in calvarial and limb development. The sensitivity of the FGF receptor 2 to mutational changes explains the phenotypic differences seen in patients with Crouzon's disease and Apert syndrome, who both possess similar allelic mutations of FGF receptor 2.

Investigators have been interested in evaluating the expression of FGF receptor 2 at the tissue level in patients with Apert syndrome. Researchers recently reported a similar study of Crouzon's patients, which suggested that the genetic mutation appeared was expressed at the tissue level. Patients with Crouzon's disease showed lower levels of FGF receptor 2 in all cranial sutures compared to nonsyndromic patients with an isolated craniosynostosis. In addition, stenosed sutures from Crouzon's patients had significantly less FGF receptor 2 staining than nonstenosed sutures from the same patients.

The results of recent investigations are similar to those reported for Crouzon's disease. The low activity of FGF receptor 2 in cranial sutures of Apert syndrome patients, as shown by specific cellular staining, suggests that the mutations occurring at the level of the FGF receptor 2 gene translate to the tissue level. Patients with Apert syndrome demonstrated significantly lower levels of FGF receptor 2 staining in cranial sutures than patients with a nonsyndromic, isolated craniosynostosis. These findings are likely due to the location of the mutation affecting FGF receptor 2 in Apert syndrome patients. Wilkie and colleagues identified specific missense substitutions involving adjacent amino acids in the linker between the second and third extracellular immunoglobulin-like domains of the FGF receptor of Apert syndrome patients. Mutations in this region affect the three-dimensional conformation of the receptor and may decrease specific anti-FGF receptor 2 antibody binding in immunochemical assays.

Adapted from S.E. White, *Cellular Biology: The Correlation of Apert Syndrome with Growth Factor Receptor Levels.* © 1997.

1. Give a title to this passage:

____

2. In your own words, what is the relationship between growth factor receptors and the syndromes mentioned in the passage?

____

____

3. What is the relationship between Apert syndrome and Crouzon's disease?

____

____

Answers to Scientific Passage Exercise 2

1. Possible titles include: Apert syndrome correlates with decreased growth factor receptor levels; Apert syndrome and Crouzon's disease correlate with decreased growth factor receptor levels.
2. Paragraph one of the passage indicates that the syndromes mentioned in the passage are linked to mutations of growth factor receptors.
3. Both of these conditions correlate with decreased levels of FGF receptor 2 in cranial sutures.

Now, on the eighth MCAT practice passage, keep in mind the speed-reading and comprehension techniques that have worked best for you so far. This passage is relatively short, but full of technical and scientific details. Try using the four steps outlined in the beginning of this chapter to help with the technical aspects of this passage. Try to identify important concepts when you skim the passage. Also, remember to define any unfamiliar words after you first skim through the passage.

Directions:
Record the times that you start and finish reading this passage in minutes and seconds. Subtract your starting time from your finishing time to find your total.

MCAT Practice Passage VIII

	Minutes	Seconds	
Your finishing time:			
Your starting time:			(subtract)
Your total time:			

Record starting time now, and begin reading.

MCAT Practice Passage VIII

Acquired Immunodeficiency Syndrome (AIDS) or the pre-AIDS condition, AIDS-Related Complex (ARC), are both due to infection by the human immunodeficiency virus (HIV). Infection with HIV is a leading cause of dementia, or loss of intellectual function, in young adults. A large proportion of patients who develop early dementia have some of a tetrad of signs known as Teshke's tetrad. These are glabellar release, snout release, slowed saccadic eye movements, and difficulty repeating numbers backwards.

The glabellar release sign is evaluated by gently tapping with a reflex hammer between the eyebrows on the forehead and looking for continuous synchronous eyelid movement. Patients are asked not to blink. Blinking after 15 taps is scored as a positive glabellar release sign. The snout release sign is similar, but involves pressing the examiner's index finger vertically against the patient's closed lips and gently tapping the index finger with a reflex hammer. Repeated pursing–pouting lip movement is considered a positive response.

Saccadic eye movements refer to slow, horizontal synchronous side-to-side movements of the eyes. These are evaluated by placing the examiner's index fingers vertically approximately 9 inches apart and 12 inches anterior to the patient's face. The patient is then asked to look from one finger to the other as rapidly as possible. Either a repeatedly prolonged delay in initiation or a slowness of eye movement is considered abnormal.

Ability to repeat numbers backward is evaluated by beginning with three numbers, then proceeding to four and five. Only after correctly repeating three numbers backward can the patient be advanced to four or five. Only patients who correctly perform five numbers backward at least once are scored as normal.

The tetrad is a valuable tool in the evaluation of early dementia in HIV-infected patients because it helps demonstrate levels of brain involvement by HIV. HIV brain disease principally involves brain white matter and subcortical structures such as the basal ganglia and thalamus. A positive glabellar response and slowed saccadic eye movements are associated with basal ganglia disease. Repetition of numbers backward tests thalamic and cortical areas. The positive snout release sign tests upper brain stem and/or its cortical connections.

When 50 normal individuals were tested for the tetrad, no one exhibited more than two abnormal responses. There were no positive snout signs, only 16% showed positive glabellar, 2% had saccadic eye slowing, and 12% had difficulty reciting numbers backward.

Conversely, once even mild HIV dementia begins, at least three of four signs are apparent. The value of the tetrad is to predict which HIV-infected patients may be developing early dementia, and to assess the level of HIV brain involvement in HIV-infected patients.

Directions:
Record the time that you finished reading in the space provided at the beginning of the passage. Subtract your starting time from your finishing time to find out how long it took you to read it.

Your reading rate is: ______________________________.

Comprehension Questions

1. Which of the following statements characterizes HIV dementia?

A. Mild HIV dementia is characterized by two of four positive Teshke tetrad signs.
B. Moderate HIV dementia is characterized by at least three of four positive Teshke tetrad signs.
C. Mild HIV dementia is characterized by at least three of four positive Teshke tetrad signs
D. Moderate HIV dementia is characterized by two of four positive Teshke tetrad signs.

2. Which of the following choices is the most accurate test of actual HIV brain involvement?

A. The snout-release sign
B. The glabellar-release sign
C. Saccadic eye movements
D. Not enough information to determine

3. Which of the following results is associated with basal ganglia disease?

A. Positive snout-release sign
B. Difficulty repeating numbers backward
C. Negative glabellar response
D. Slowed saccadic eye movements

4. Which of the following statements is false?

A. Repeating five or more numbers backward is considered normal.
B. A negative glabellar release sign is associated with blinking before 15 taps.
C. Slowed vertical eye movements or difficulty initiating these movements is scored as a positive saccadic eye movement sign.
D. The basal ganglia and thalamus are considered subcortical structures.

5. Consider the following statement: Snout release is a more primitive reflex than glabellar release because snout release involves the brain stem, whereas glabellar release involves the basal ganglia.

A. The statement is supported by the passage.
B. The statement is contradicted by the passage.
C. The statement is neither supported nor contradicted by the passage.
D. Not enough information to determine.

6. A patient is administered all the Teshke's tetrad signs. The patient blinks 12 times, purses and pouts, has normal side-to-side eye movements, and can correctly repeat only three numbers backward.

A. This patient has only two positive tetrad signs.
B. This patient has only three positive tetrad signs.
C. This patient has only one positive tetrad sign.
D. This patient has three negative tetrad signs.

7. Which of the following statements is LEAST supported by information given in the passage?

A. A patient who blinks 10 times in response to glabellar-release sign stimulation is considered to have absence of the glabellar-release sign.
B. A demented patient who demonstrates positive responses to all of Teshke's tetrad is infected with HIV.
C. The value of the tetrad is to help physicians predict which HIV-infected patients may be going on to develop HIV dementia.
D. Normal patients, without evidence of HIV infection, would be unlikely to demonstrate more than one or two positive responses if given the Teshke's tetrad test.

Directions:
Correct your answers by using the answer key at the end of this chapter. Allow 12.5 percentage points for each correct answer.

MCAT Practice Passage VIII Comprehension Score and Reading Rate

Your comprehension test score ___________%. *Your reading rate* ____________________.

Discussion of MCAT Practice Passage VIII

This is another expository passage; it defines Teshke's tetrad and tells why it is important to determine whether a patient responds to the tetrad. The first paragraph introduces Teshke's tetrad as indicative of a set of symptoms of HIV-induced dementia. The next three paragraphs explain the tetrad: glabellar-release signs, saccadic eye movements, and the inability to repeat numbers backward beginning by threes and proceeding to fours and fives. After drawing out for the reader what the tetrad consists of, the fifth paragraph explains why it is important to look at this tetrad. Paragraph six gives evidence that healthy adults have few occurrences of responses to this tetrad, and the final paragraph explains that the percentage of responses to this tetrad increases when HIV is present. Remember that the passages in the MCAT Verbal Reasoning test discuss many different fields, and a wide variety of information will be covered. **All the information you will need to answer the questions will be contained in the passage.**

Answers and Explanations to MCAT Passage VIII

1. **C** Solve this question by evaluating each answer choice carefully. Note that each answer choice mentions the Teshke tetrad of signs. Look for the paragraph that discusses HIV dementia and the Teshke signs. The last paragraph of this passage states that patients with HIV dementia demonstrate at least three of the four signs, which supports choice C.

2. **D** There are several important key words in this question. The words *most accurate* and *actual* are very important in this question. You should look for tests that accurately evaluate actual HIV brain involvement. After a quick review of the passage, it is clear that the passage does not state which method is most accurate. Eliminate choices A, B, and C because they are not supported by the passage. This question was designed to see if you overconclude and arrive at answers based on speculation.
3. **D** Start by finding the paragraph that discusses basal ganglia disease. The fifth paragraph discusses basal ganglia disease. As discussed in the paragraph, slowed saccadic eye movements are associated with basal ganglia disease. However, note that the passage does not imply a cause of basal ganglia disease.
4. **C** Consider the validity of each choice. Eliminate the choices that are true statements. The fourth paragraph supports choice A as a correct statement. The second paragraph validates that choice B is true. The second sentence of the fifth paragraph indicates that both the basal ganglia and thalamus are subcortical structures; therefore, eliminate choice D. Based on the process of elimination, the correct answer must be choice C. Also, the third paragraph defines an abnormal or positive saccadic eye movement sign as being an inability to perform or initiate horizontal (not vertical) eye movements.
5. **C** The question stem presents a conclusion. You must evaluate this conclusion to see if it is supported. Begin your evaluation by checking if the passage discusses which reflexes are most primitive. Note that the passage does not allow you to reach the conclusion given in the question stem because the passage does not discuss which areas of the brain or which reflexes are more primitive. Because the information you need to evaluate the statement is unavailable, the statement is neither supported nor contradicted by the passage.
6. **A** The patient blinks only 12 times, so this is a negative, or normal, response. The patient purses and pouts, so this is a positive, or abnormal, response. The patient has normal side-to-side movements; thus, saccadic eye movements are normal. Because the patient can only repeat three numbers backward, this response is abnormal. In total, the patient has two positive and two negative tetrad signs.

   Choices B, C, and D are false, because they incorrectly state the number of positive or negative tetrad signs.
7. **B** Eliminate choices that appear to be supported by information contained in the passage. Identify the choice that is supported to the least degree or the choice that is not supported at all. Choice A appears supported. The second paragraph indicates that blinking 15 times is scored as a positive glabellar sign. You can infer that blinking less than 15 times is most likely a negative test result. Choice C is supported by the first sentence in the fifth paragraph. Choice D is a reasonable statement and is generally supported by statements made throughout the passage. Choice B is the least supported. Both the fifth and the last paragraphs discuss the tetrad and HIV. Although the tetrad demonstrates brain involvement in HIV-infected patients, the passage does not state that the tetrad proves HIV infection.

Chapter 10

Review Exercises and Practice Verbal Reasoning Passages

The best way to increase your reading speed and comprehension is to **practice.** In this chapter, you will find a set of skill-building drills and MCAT Verbal Reasoning passages with comprehension questions. The drills are included as exercises to help you review the speed-reading and comprehension techniques you learned throughout this book. In Chapter 11, three full-length practice Verbal Reasoning tests are provided for additional practice.

By now, you have discovered techniques introduced in this guide that work best for you. Always remember these basic concepts:

1. Concentrate on **speed.** Comprehension will follow.
2. **Do not get distracted.**
3. **Do not read word-for-word** at first—concentrate on the meaning of the whole passage.
4. **Keep moving**—do not stop for too long on any question or section of a passage.
5. **Keep your goal in mind**—complete the section in less than 85 minutes, so that you will have time to go back and answer any difficult questions that you skipped. This gives you approximately 9 minutes per passage.
6. **Concentrate!** As always, be an **active reader.**

Here are some additional exercises to solidify your new speed-reading and comprehension skills. Practice your new skills as often as you can on your textbooks and other class reading, as well as newspapers, magazines, and other publications you read every day.

Review Exercises

Comprehension, Skimming, and Titling

Quickly skim this paragraph, looking only for the main idea.

> Probably the best known, most prolific, and most versatile of North African writers to use the French language is Mohammed Dib. An Algerian, he was brought up in a strongly Muslim-influenced atmosphere. Both Arabic and French were his native languages, but he chose to write most of his journalistic works, books, poems, and plays in French. His work presents itself as a more penetrating investigation of the human being as much in reference to Algerian terror as renewed insight into the dilemmas of the Algerian people and humans the world over. Dib worked as a journalist the early part of his career, then published *La Grande Maison* (The Big House). The central character is Omar, who is a child at the beginning of the book and whom we see grow through the course of the narrative. He ponders his role in the activities of which he is a part, gaining occasional insights into an altered future. This is an analogy for the feelings between Algeria and France, expressed originally and sensitively by Dib, yet "boldly accusing."

Quick!

The main idea of the this passage:

____

A title for this passage:

____

Identifying the Thesis

Quickly find the thesis sentence in the following paragraph:

Although democracy may seem to be the ultimate solution to the political problems of the world, many countries have succeeded through noncompetitive regimes. In such systems, selection of the political elite is a narrow, highly selective process. However, a limited sort of pluralism exists in the upper strata of these political machines, as demonstrated in countries such as Mexico and Russia. It is possible for those who adhere to political guidelines to reach the top in these two countries, but generally a different sort of person characterizes the political elite in either country. Mexico tends to favor highly educated, trained personnel, whereas Russia leans towards the experienced and above-all loyal politician who has proven himself on the political battleground.

The thesis of this paragraph:

____

Skimming

Quickly skim this paragraph for the main idea:

When a xxxxx being is x part of x corporate body, that human xxxxx loses his xx her human individuality and xxxxxxx as x cell is in x larger body. The xxxxx acts as xx agent for xxx owners or stockholders of xxx corporation, and he xx she xxxx abide by their wishes xxx decisions. xxxx is the nature of the free market—stockholders express xxxxx approval xxx a business's products and practices xx purchasing stock; the marketplace expresses its xxxxxxxx by purchasing xxx company's products. Both stockholders and consumers are and should xx free xx take their business xxxxxxxxx. The corporation itself, xx the midst xx these market forces, has xxx responsibility only xx increase xxx xxxxxxx by selling more of the product, raising its xxxxxx, increasing efficiency xx xxx production, lowering wages, xx whatever xxxx the market will bear.

Restate the main idea of this paragraph:

____

Scanning

Circle the word that means **almost the same** as the first word in each line. Go as fast as you can, timing yourself. See if you can do them all in 45 seconds.

1.	huge	improper immense immoral impute impure
2.	dense	society song sock solid sop sojourn solo
3.	covenant	pack pork polo pact pacify paper pad
4.	falter	red reel rake rickets rifle right rope robe
5.	departure	end endorse exit enrage exude exult
6.	health	veil vehicle value vanish vigor varnish
7.	rapture	jingle jewelry joint jump jiggle joy
8.	shake	title toad toast treat trowel tremor tricycle
9.	fast	stick stink starve save shave shawl shake
10.	acute	critical criticize cryptic cry cracker crow
11.	prune	trick trim trip trickle trek trellis trinket trench
12.	mimic	imprint impress imitate immoral inflate infamous

Time ____________

Answers to Scanning Drill

1. immense
2. solid
3. pact
4. reel
5. exit
6. vigor
7. joy
8. tremor
9. starve
10. critical
11. trim
12. imitate

Reading for Key Words

Underline the key words in the following paragraph.

The movement to improve the education of middle-class girls in Victorian England brought with it many debates and criticisms. The traditional place for the female was in the home, caring for children, running the house, and providing companionship for husbands or fathers. Girls were taught primarily in the home until the late nineteenth century, when the Education Act of 1870 was passed. After 1870, girls' schools were gradually established, but while the quality of education they received improved steadily as time went by, anything but the most basic education was met with great opposition.

Marking a Text and Reading Unfamiliar Material

Practice marking while reading this passage. Remember the marking symbols (see Table 6-1). Also, remember to skim difficult material first before marking it up.

Sandpiles, vortices in superconductors, nonlinear electronic circuits, and lightning discharges are all examples of systems characterized by many interacting moving objects that are pushed towards instability by an external force. Through experiments, computer simulations, and theoretical work on avalanches and instabilities in such systems, University of Michigan physics professors Franco Nori, Michael Bretz, and Stuart Field have spent the past few years investigating the intricate transport phenomena, from very slow motion to sudden bursts, observed as these systems are driven toward marginally stable states by external forces.

With Bretz's focus on sandpiles and other granular materials, Field's work on nonlinear electronic circuits and superconductors, and Nori's theoretical work—both analytical and computational—they have put themselves at the forefront of the new wave of interest in instabilities in complex systems. Their work involves computer-assisted imaging of avalanches in sand, analysis of water-droplet avalanches falling off a continuously sprayed Plexiglas dome, instabilities in electronic circuits, studies of granular material in rotating drums, onset of electron motion in semiconductors, and several studies of the avalanche-like behavior of vortices as they move through superconducting material. In each of these systems, an externally applied force slowly drives the system to a "threshold of instability" and unstable state where particle transport occurs in the form of an avalanche, which releases energy and allows the system to return to a more stable configuration.

Adapted from "Modern Physics News" © 1994.

Practice MCAT Verbal Reasoning Passages

The MCAT Verbal Reasoning test is the first section of the MCAT and is 85 minutes long. You must be able to read nine passages of 500–600 words in length each, and answer 6–10 multiple-choice questions about each passage in the time allotted. There will be a total of 65 questions. Thus, this gives you about 9 minutes to read each passage and answer questions about it. Broken down, this means you must be able to skim the question stems and read a passage in 3–4 minutes. This gives you 5 minutes to answer the questions. You must work fast in order to complete the Verbal Reasoning test.

In order to help you practice the strategies discussed in this guide, a set of practice passages is provided. This set of passages allows you to work on your timing. This drill consists of three passages, each followed by a set of about eight questions. On your timer, give yourself 27 minutes to complete the section.

For this drill, use the following steps and strategies that have been emphasized in this book:

1. **Skim the questions first,** but ignore answer choices. This will give you an idea of what is important in the passage. Use no more than 20–30 seconds for this step.
2. **Try to preview and read each passage in about 2½ minutes.** Remember to use the strategies discussed in previous chapters. Mark the text appropriately.
3. **Proceed to answering questions.** Feel free to look back in the passage for answers to questions. Hopefully, you will have marked important areas in the passage to help yourself quickly find answers.

Directions:
Record the times that you start and finish reading this practice MCAT Verbal Reasoning passage in minutes and seconds. Subtract your starting time from your finishing time to find your total.

MCAT Practice Verbal Reasoning Section

	Minutes	Seconds	
Your finishing time:			
Your starting time:			(subtract)
Your total time:			

Record starting time now, and begin reading.

Passage IX (Questions 1–8)

If ever there were a man's world, it seems the Navy is it. Women in the Navy have long been a problematic, and even controversial minority. Although still not permitted officially to fly or to serve in combat missions, women have come to occupy an uncomfortable place in this man's world. While "women's place" in this world has long been debated by men, women themselves have just begun to make their presence in this debate felt publicly.

In the wake of the Anita Hill, Clarence Thomas hearings, women in many different "men's worlds" have begun to speak up about sexual harassment and sexual assault in the workplace. Women lawyers, waitresses, business people, teachers, doctors, nurses, and secretaries have come to understand that many of the minor and major grievances they have about work are legally defined as sexual harassment. While these women certainly did not need a legal code to feel abused, knowing that they might be able to make a case in court has empowered many women and given them a voice to complain with. This year women in the Navy joined the ranks of those women who definitely have something to fight about.

At the 1991 Tailhook convention, several incidents occurred which brought sexual harassment and sexual discrimination in the Navy to the attention of the public. At the same convention at which a woman pilot was booed and hissed at by her comrades for asking nine male admirals when women pilots would be able to fly combat missions, a woman helicopter pilot was groped and grabbed by a gauntlet of male officers. Both incidents seemed meant to shame women in the Navy, reinforcing dramatically that many men would like to see the Navy remain a man's world.

The incident in which the woman was groped triggered a Defense Department criminal investigation, stirred up official concern in the White House, voiced by the President, and led to the resignation of Navy Secretary H. Lawrence Garrett III. Despite Garrett's dramatic resignation, which he hoped would send a strong message to Navy officers that sexual harassment was intolerable, and help settle the controversy, many men and women agree that the Navy has a long way to go to rid its institutions of sexual discrimination.

Much of the debate revolves around the question of women in combat. Many women feel that they will not be considered truly equal until they are allowed to participate on an equal basis with men in combat. Several women officers claim that "separate" can never be "equal." Arguments against women in combat generally appeal to the potential for sexual attraction and distraction in critical combat scenes. It would appear that many men don't trust themselves or their male colleagues when a woman is around. Few actually question the competency of their female counterparts.

Some of the male officers who would like to see women in combat admit to feelings of resentment when they are sent away from family and friends in missions, while their female comrades stay home. Many women officers recognize their resentment and claim that it only heightens the potential for misunderstanding between the sexes and sexual harassment.

From R. Heftel, *Inequalities and the Navy: A Study*. © 1997.

1. This essay assumes a link between:

A. Anita Hill, Clarence Thomas, and the Navy.
B. the Hill–Thomas hearings and the Navy.
C. the Hill–Thomas hearings and women's incentive to talk about sexual harassment.
D. Clarence Thomas and sexual harassment.

2. The author of this article would most likely define a "man's world" as a place in which:

I. there are mostly men.
II. men have most of the power.
III. women complain.

A. I, II, and III only
B. I only
C. I and III only
D. I and II only

3. Many women in the Navy want to participate in combat missions because they:

A. are macho.
B. want a chance to prove themselves.
C. want to be treated equally.
D. are brave.

4. Some men in the Navy would like to see women in combat because:

A. it would be fair.
B. they miss their wives.
C. combat is lonely.
D. combat is prestigious.

5. According to this article, many who oppose women in combat argue that women are too:

A. weak.
B. demanding.
C. pretty.
D. ignorant.

6. One might infer from the passage that legal authority is to confidence as:

A. equality:respect.
B. combat:competency.
C. the Navy:sexual harassment.
D. Anita Hill:sexual harassment.

7. According to the article, Navy Secretary H. Lawrence Garrett, III resigned because he was:

A. threatened.
B. ridiculed.
C. frightened.
D. appalled.

8. The passage seems to assume that sexual harassment is the result of:

A. ignorant male aggression.
B. inequality based on sex.
C. minority rule.
D. male hormones.

Passage X (Questions 9–16)

In my seventh grade science class, each student was required to do an oral presentation based on individual research collected over the course of the semester. I remember being very scared when it was my turn to present my findings on the migration patterns of the monarch butterfly. I had anticipated the 10-minute presentation for weeks. I made colorful visual aids and practiced my talk at least a hundred times. When the moment actually came, my brain seemed to float outside my body. I could hear my voice in the room, but couldn't connect what I heard with the labored maneuverings of my pasty mouth. When I was done, the class applauded and Ms. Malone complimented me on my drawings of flying butterflies. I was a success, and gradually my brain came back to my body.

Two weeks later, as I was relaxing and coasting through the rest of the semester, Bobby Shank gave his presentation on black holes. He was very enthusiastic, and if his brain was floating outside his body, he certainly didn't let on. What was supposed to be a 10-minute presentation lasted over half an hour. Several students began to shift restlessly in their chairs as he breached the 25-minute mark, but I remained fairly interested in what this normally shy kid was getting all excited about. He was telling tales of lost space ships, alien creatures, and inverted galaxies. At half past the hour, Mark Banter became agitated and started yelling, "They don't exist." And still louder, "It's just a hypothesis. They don't exist." "Black holes are an invention of science fiction." "You can't prove they exist." Bobby said, "Yes they do," finished his presentation abruptly, and went back to his seat in the middle of the room. Ms. Malone thanked Bobby and the class applauded nervously. We were all let out early for lunch.

I hadn't thought about Bobby Shank for years until I recently picked up an old issue of *Scientific American*. Years after Bobby's fateful talk, it seems scientists are considering seriously the possibility that a black hole exists at the center of our universe. No one appears to be talking specifically about lost space ships and alien creatures, but mention has been made of a collapsed mass of about three million stars in the middle of the Milky Way.

Although Bobby may have relied a little too heavily on science fiction novels for his facts, general relativity, as theorized by Einstein, does allow for the possibility of collapsed mass dense enough to stop everything, including light, from escaping its gravitational pull. Black holes are nearly impossible objects to study, as they are invisible, and though able to suck great masses into their realms, the emit no radiation. Scientists now believe, however, that while radiation cannot be emitted from a black hole itself, it might be traced from material as it falls into a black hole. Thus the effects of a black hole, if not the black hole itself, might be studied.

I imagine it will be a long time before anyone knows for sure whether or not a black hole keeps our galaxy in motion, but Bobby Shank may have been onto something back in the seventh grade. I hope Mark Banter stumbles across the article I found sometime before our next high school reunion. Whether or not black holes do exist, a galactic wrong needs to be righted in the Milky Way.

By M. Elliot. *Bobby Shank May Have Known.*

9. The purpose of this passage is to:

A. educate.
B. confuse.
C. remember.
D. entertain.

10. The information the author cites about the existence of black holes is:

A. conclusive.
B. fictional.
C. possible.
D. ridiculous.

11. The author of this passage is ultimately most concerned with:

A. scientific fact.
B. social relations.
C. pedagogy.
D. human physiology.

12. How could black holes be studied?

A. They cannot be studied.
B. Through hard work
C. No one knows.
D. Indirectly

13. Black holes are:

I. the subject of science fiction novels.
II. invisible.
III. like inescapable vacuums.

A. II and III only
B. I, II, and III
C. I and II only
D. II only

14. The author of the passage probably writes:

A. for *Scientific American*.
B. for the *Wall Street Journal*.
C. poetry.
D. short stories.

15. The author of the passage once felt her brain was floating outside her body because she:

A. forgot her speech.
B. was nervous.
C. was successful.
D. was over prepared.

16. When Bobby Shank gave his presentation in the seventh grade, the author of this passage:

A. knew black holes did not exist.
B. loved science fiction.
C. was curious.
D. was bored.

Passage XI (Questions 17–24)

Although it still looks like rock and roll is here to stay, rock's once culturally explosive, disruptive power appears to have been taken over in the last decade by rap. Rap music has become the confrontational form that everyone—including politicians—wants to argue about. Politicians from both major political parties have made strong statements about rap music. Vocal politicians who have confronted this controversial issue include Bill Clinton and Robert Dole. Both of these men have been critical of various components of rap and have directed criticism at specific artists in the rap music scene. It is interesting that these two politicians come from different support bases and claim to have different views on social issues.

When President Clinton criticized rapper and political activist Sister Souljah for remarks she made in the *Washington Post* concerning race and violence, he threw a very articulate young woman into the public spotlight, and got people across the country talking about the politics of rap music with increased fervor. While Clinton and other white politicians claim to seek an end to racial division, rap, one of the country's most popular music forms, seems to advocate racial division and violence to many listeners. The issues here are clouded. Is the criticism of rap based on the verbal content of the music, or one of racial bias and an attempt to control a culture trying to express itself?

Bob Dole also created much public debate and controversy when he criticized rap as a contributing force to youth violence and antisocial behavior. However, Dole has not limited his comments to rap. He has also been critical of some forms of rock music and has directed criticism at numerous major motion pictures. Dole's focus appeared to be directed at the media in general. He has both stated and implied that the entertainment industry has been irresponsible in marketing music, film, and television programs that emphasize sex and violence.

According to John Leland of *Newsweek*, music and other popular cultural forms act as symbolic terrain upon which various different societal fears and fantasies can be enacted. Leland claims that while rock and roll and rap have both represented symbolic territory between blacks and whites in the United States, they have mapped different fears and fantasies. If rock and roll was a stand-in for interracial sex, rap is a stand-in for interracial violence.

In attempting to explain the popularity of rap music with white audiences, Leland says that rap offers listeners a neat, clean, controlled medium on which to explore messy, ugly fears and realities. The problem with these tidy explorations through music lyrics, however, is that they also allow white listeners to feel they are confronting racism and violence without really doing anything. Many white listeners feel much more comfortable interacting with their CD players than with their black neighbors.

Although all rap artists are not black, "blackness" has become the identifying mark of this music form. Crystallized into the most salient characteristic of rap music by the group Public Enemy, according to John Leland, "blackness" is the sign that rap artists, including white rappers, must somehow construct in order to be successful. White rappers try to promote their "authenticity" by surrounding themselves with black performers or by talking about their childhood growing up in "black neighborhoods."

MTV is perhaps the medium most directly responsible for the growing white interest in rap music. MTV hosts special rap programs for its mostly white audience. It is interesting to note that when MTV first started, it would rarely show the video of a black artist. MTV is now finding that black culture sells to its white audience. Again, the nature of the relationship this represents is a problematic one that does not necessarily promote any cross-cultural understanding or any action on the part of white viewers. If black culture sells to a white audience on MTV, it sells as a contained package and allows its white viewers to participate in a touristic voyeurism. And when the music program is over, white viewers can go back to a world in which they do not necessarily have to think about racism and violence.

Rap may communicate a different message to its black listeners. Many rappers say that they predicted events such as the Los Angeles uprising years ago and talked about them in their lyrics. Others have called rap the best news source for black Americans. And still others have cited rap music as a means of instructional socialization for young black children. Whatever it may mean to its various listeners, it looks like rap music is here to stay.

Adapted from L.R. Nelson. *Rap: What does it Mean?* © 1996. Rolling Stone Magazine.

17. According to the passage, white audiences often use listening to rap music as a substitute for:

A. talking to black people.
B. racism.
C. sex.
D. rock and roll.

18. Based on the passage, John Leland might say that music is a kind of:

A. trickery.
B. delusion.
C. theater.
D. opiate.

19. For the white audience, how is rap often treated?

A. As a commodity
B. As an adventure
C. As a bargain
D. As a decoy

20. Politicians are talking about rap music because it corresponds to:

A. popularity.
B. entertainment.
C. fantasies.
D. race relations.

21. According to information given in the passage, which of the following statements best explains why MTV shows rap videos?

A. To educate white audiences
B. To attract black audiences
C. To be politically correct
D. To make money

22. Which statement describes rap music?

I. It causes racial violence.
II. It depicts racial violence.
III. It means different things to different listeners.

A. I, II, and III
B. II and III only
C. I and II only
D. I and III only

23. One can infer from the passage that when rock and roll was becoming popular:

A. everyone was having sex.
B. society was less violent.
C. people feared interracial sex.
D. there was no interracial violence.

24. At one time, rock and roll was:

A. disliked.
B. controversial.
C. violent.
D. disdained.

Directions:
Correct your answers by using the answer key. Allow 2.5 percentage points for each correct answer. A comprehension score in the 80%–85% range corresponds to a score of 10 or better (top 20th percentile).

MCAT Practice Section Comprehension Score and Reading Rate

Your comprehension test score ____________%. *Your reading rate* ____________

Answers and Explanations to MCAT Practice Verbal Reasoning Section

1. **C** This question asks you to identify the assumed link between the main persons and events described in the passage. In the first sentence of paragraph two, the link is exposed. The paragraph points out that in the wake of the Hill–Thomas hearings, women are beginning to speak up about sexual harassment.
2. **D** Independently evaluate each of the statements. Identify the statements you believe are true, and eliminate answer choices that do not contain the true statements. Paragraph one supports the first statement. The passage emphasizes institutions, such as the Navy, which typically have few women. The entire passage is about power and equality, validating statement II. Statement III is not well supported; the passage infers that until recently, women do not necessarily complain in male-dominated places.
3. **C** Choice A is a humorous, unsupported choice that you can quickly eliminate. Although choice B may be a true statement, it is not specifically mentioned in the passage. Choice D is an overgeneralization that may be true in some cases, but it is not discussed in the passage. Choice C is supported directly in paragraph five.
4. **A** The first sentence of paragraph six suggests that some male officers in the Navy would like to see women in combat to equalize the feelings that arise from being separated from family. Choice B is incorrect because it describes how some men in the Navy feel about being separated from family; it does not answer the question being asked. Choice C is speculative and not discussed in the passage. Choice D is completely unsupported.
5. **C** Identify the section of the passage that discusses women in combat. Paragraph five deals with the subject of women in combat. The paragraph indicates that some men fear that their attraction for women comrades will distract them in combat. Look at the choices carefully, and select the choice that is most closely related to male attraction and distraction by women.
6. **A** This question presents a work pair and asks you to select an answer choice with a similar relationship between work pairs. The question stem presents the words *legal authority* and *confidence*. Note that confidence is most likely dependent on legal authority. It is less likely that legal authority would depend on confidence. Select the word pair among the choices in which the second word depends on the first. Choice A is a reasonable choice. Respect may be dependent on equality. Choices B, C, and D are less likely choices. Competency is probably not dependent on combat. Sexual harassment is not dependent on the Navy or Anita Hill.
7. **D** The answer is discussed in paragraph four. The Navy Secretary resigned in order to send a strong message to officers that sexual harassment is unacceptable. You must choose the most likely reason why he resigned. Choices A and B are an unlikely choices. There is no evidence in the passage that the Navy Secretary was either threatened or ridiculed. In addition, the fourth paragraph does not indicate that anything frightened the Navy Secretary. Phrases such as "dramatic resignation" and "harassment was intolerable" suggest that the Navy Secretary was surprised and shocked by the exhibited behaviors. Choice D best describes the reason why the Navy Secretary resigned.
8. **B** It is easy to eliminate all three of the incorrect choices. Choice A is not supported by the passage because the causes for the harassment are not discussed. In addition, the passage does not strongly label anyone as ignorant. Choice C is incorrect because the passage does not state that the minority (women) rule the Navy. Choice D is not implied or stated. Therefore, by process of elimination, choice B is the best answer.

9. **D** This passage has a light and humorous tone. It is much easier to read than most MCAT-style passages because it tells a story. The passage is not informative about any topic in particular, so eliminate choice A. The passage is neither confusing nor difficult to recall, so eliminate choices B and C.
10. **C** Look for evidence in the passage that supports the existence of black holes. Paragraph three discusses this topic. The author states, "scientists are considering seriously the possibility that a black hole exists." This statement directly supports choice C. The passage does not indicate that the existence of black holes is conclusive (choice A). Paragraph three also gives enough credibility to black holes to eliminate choices B and D.
11. **B** This passage tells a story, and it is not a scientific or fact-based passage. Therefore, eliminate choice A. Pedagogy implies education or schooling. Choice C is an unlikely choice because the author does not discuss the issue of education to any significant degree. Choice D is completely unsupported by the passage. Choice B is the best choice. The author appears concerned mostly with social relations and the relationship between the characters described in the passage. For example, the final paragraph emphasizes that Bobby Shank may have been on to something and that Mark Banter may have been wrong in condemning Bobby's presentation.
12. **D** Paragraph four discusses black holes and current scientific beliefs. Note an important phrase in paragraph four: ". . .the effect of black holes, if not black holes themselves, can be studied." This phrase implies that if black holes cannot be studied, perhaps the effects of the black holes can. This implication supports choice D. Choice A can be eliminated because the passage indicates that black holes may be studied. Choice B is speculative and not supported by evidence from the passage. Choice C is contradicted by the previously quoted phrase, which indicates that the effects of black holes may be studied.
13. **B** Refer to paragraph four, which provides information about black holes. Note that all three statements are directly supported by this paragraph. Thus, choice B (statements I, II, and III) is the best answer.
14. **D** Use inference to select the best answer choice. You can infer from the tone that this passage is more like a short story than a scientific article or a serious informational piece. Therefore, you can eliminate choices A and B. There is no poetry in the passage, so choice C is unlikely.
15. **B** Find the paragraph in the passage that discusses "floating outside the body." Note that this is discussed in the first paragraph. The author implies in the first paragraph that she was scared to give a presentation, which supports choice B. There is no evidence that the author forgot her speech (choice A). Although the author's speech appears successful, this is not a reason why the author felt her brain floating outside the body; thus, eliminate choice C. The passage does not imply that the author was overprepared (choice D).
16. **C** In paragraph two the author states that she remained fairly interested in what Bobby Shank had to say about black holes, which is most consistent with choice C. Choice A is incorrect because the author never indicates that she knew black holes did not exist. Choice B can be eliminated because it is speculative and unsupported by the passage. Choice D is contradicted by paragraph two.
17. **A** Paragraph four describes John Leland's hypotheses as they relate to rap music and white audiences. Leland suggests that white audiences may be more comfortable listening to the work of black musicians than interacting with their black neighbors. The passage does not suggest that white audiences listen to rap music as a substitute for racism (choice B), sex (choice C), or rock and roll (choice D).

18. **C** This question requires that you use inference to predict what John Leland might say. Focus on the paragraphs of the passage that discuss Leland's philosophies. In particular, note paragraph three. The first sentence of this paragraph uses metaphorical language. Leland states that music and other cultural forms act as terrains, where fears and fantasies can be enacted. Note that Leland uses theatrical terms, such as *act* and *enacted*. This supports choice C. Leland does not suggest that music is a kind of trickery (choice A) or delusion (choice B). Choice D is also incorrect because Leland does not imply that music causes euphoria or is addictive like an opiate.
19. **A** This question can be answered from information contained in paragraph six. As discussed in this paragraph, MTV often offers rap and black culture as a "contained package" to its white audience. Choice A, or a commodity, best describes a "contained package."
20. **D** The second paragraph discusses politicians and rap music. The paragraph states that many white politicians claim to seek an end to racial division. Thus, politicians are likely talking about rap music because it has ties to race relations. Although rap music may be popular, the passage does not infer that politicians are talking about rap because it corresponds to popularity (choice A). Similarly, there is no link between rap discussions and politicians and entertainment (choice B) or fantasies (choice C).
21. **D** The passage states in paragraph six that rap videos "sell." This supports the statement in choice D. Choice D is a better selection than the other choices because it is directly supported by statements in the passage. Choice A may be a correct statement, but it is not the best answer. Although white audiences may be educated by rap videos, the passage does not imply that education is the goal of MTV. Similarly, choice B may be a correct statement, but it is not discussed in the passage. Choice C is speculative and not directly supported.
22. **B** Statements II and III are supported by the passage. Paragraph three supports that rap music depicts racial violence. Paragraph seven suggests that rap music means different things to different listeners. Evaluate statement I carefully. Note that this is an emphatic statement. Recall that these are frequently incorrect responses on the Verbal Reasoning test. Statement I is not supported by the passage. It is not stated that rap music is a cause of racial violence.
23. **C** Answer this question after evaluating paragraph three, which deals with rock and roll's effect on society. The societal fear enacted via rock and roll was interracial sex. Choices A, B, and D are unsupported statements.
24. **B** In the first paragraph, rock is described as being "culturally explosive" and "disruptive" in the past. Evaluate the choices carefully to see which word best describes how rock was perceived in the past. "Culturally explosive" is not necessarily a negative description of rock and roll. "Disruptive" does carry a negative connotation. Choices A and D may be eliminated because these are definitely negative descriptions. *Disdained* and *disliked* are synonyms. Choice C is also a negative word. In addition, the passage does not indicate that rock and roll was violent. Choice B is the best choice. *Controversial* could carry a negative or positive meaning and best describes the terms "culturally explosive" and "disruptive."

Conclusion

Regular practice is essential if you want to read quickly and efficiently. Keep up with your practice every day while you are studying for the MCAT, and review this book regularly. Also, get into the habit of reading the newspaper every day, so you can practice scanning, skimming, searching for main ideas, and quick comprehension. Challenge yourself as much as possible to be an **active** reader. Constantly ask yourself questions about **everything** you read; be critical of all your reading material. When you are done reading, tell yourself or write down what you learned and what questions you still have about the topic.

In Chapter 11, you will have a chance to put it all together and work through practice Verbal Reasoning tests. These practice tests will give you the opportunity to experience the length, difficulty, and fatigue factor associated with full-length Verbal Reasoning testing. Be sure to apply the strategies and skills that you learned in the first 10 chapters of this book. Best wishes, and here's to Verbal Reasoning success!

Chapter 11

VERBAL REASONING PRACTICE TEST 1

Suggested Time: 85 minutes

Directions: There are nine reading passages in the Verbal Reasoning test. Each passage is followed by several questions. After reading a passage, select one best answer to each question. If you are not certain of an answer, eliminate the alternatives that you know to be incorrect, and then select an answer from the remaining alternatives.

Passage I (Questions 1–7)

Russia's participation in World War I was self-contradictory, both in motives and goals. The war aims of Russia were actually to gain the Turkish Straits, Galicia, and Armenia, although the European powers felt Russia wished for world domination. As one of the great powers, Russia could not help participating in the scramble of the advanced, European, capitalist countries, just as in the preceding epoch, she could not help introducing industrialization and modernization.

The army of Tsarist Russia appeared to be unconquerable in the eyes of the common Russian peasant. However, to military analysts at the time, the army of the Tzar was a serious force only against semibarbaric people, small neighbors, and disintegrating states. In the European arena, the army could act only as part of a coalition. In the matter of Russian defense, the army could fulfill its task of protection only by recruiting the help of the vastness of Russia itself. The impassability of the roads to those unaccustomed to them and the harshness of the climate to foreign intruders made the Russian army appear stronger than it was. Additional weaknesses in the Russian army included poor communication between the commanding staff and the foot soldier and a distrust between army officers and common soldiers. This distrust was based on the differences in social class between the officers and enlisted men. The commanding staff were members of the ruling classes and the bourgeoisie, whereas common foot soldiers were peasant and serfs.

The first days of Russian battle in the war were a disgrace. Several offensives failed in rapid succession. By the spring of 1915, the Tsarist forces were in retreat. The generals took out their own criminal incapacity on the peaceful population. Enormous tracts of land were violently laid to waste. Clouds of human locusts were driven to the rear with whips. The external rout was completed with an internal one.

The War Minister summarized for his colleagues the situation at the front with these words: "I trust the impenetrable spaces of the mother land, the snow and mud, and the mercy of Saint Nicholas Mirlikisky, the Protector of Holy Russia." However, after suffering additional retreats in the battles of the next several weeks, the War Minister stated, "the present-day demands of military technique are beyond us. We simply cannot keep up with the enemy, for we are in no condition to do anything; even the new methods of warfare become causes for our failure." What the Russian generals did in response to the early losses to the enemy was unforgivable. The generals, in swift order, plugged all cracks with new human mobilizations. This created "columns of figures," when columns of fighters were really needed. About

15 million men were mobilized, and they brimmed the depots, barracks, points of transit, and battlefields. All in all, over 5 million soldiers were wounded, captured, or killed in early battles. These Russian losses were vast and tragic, yet carefully thought out to put at risk only the least important members of Tsarist society.

Adapted from Leon Trotsky, *Tsarist Russia in the War.* © 1960 by University Press.

1. The passage suggests that the Tsarist army's strength was:

A. tested and unsurpassed.
B. unknown and unrecognized.
C. predictable and moderate.
D. inflated and overestimated.

2. Based on information given in the passage, the term "human locusts" best depicts:

A. Tsarist generals.
B. enemy soldiers.
C. Russian bourgeoisie.
D. Russian peasants.

3. Which of the following statements would be most consistent with the author's view of Tsarist Russia?

A. There were great divides between the different levels of Tsarist Russian society.
B. The bourgeoisie were responsible for the injustices committed against peasants.
C. The Russian army was an extension of Tsarist limitations.
D. Russian leadership was consumed with European values.

4. The tone of the author is best described as:

A. supportive.
B. descriptive.
C. critical.
D. analytical.

5. In response to early battle losses, Russian generals employed a battle strategy based on:

A. well-trained and equipped soldiers.
B. a multifaceted attack by Russian forces.
C. modern techniques of warfare.
D. sheer numbers of soldiers.

6. Based on the passage, the picture painted for Tsarist Russia is one of:

A. class distinction.
B. equal opportunity for all.
C. economic depression.
D. a monarchy unable to control the military.

7. The passage suggests that Russian involvement in the war:

A. could have been prevented.
B. was provoked.
C. led to political upheaval.
D. could not have been helped.

Passage II (Questions 8–15)

Although a practical, affordable commercial color photographic process was not invented until the twentieth century, experimenters in photography were working to reproduce color images from the very beginning of photographic science. Commercially available color images in the nineteenth century were generally black-and-white photographs that were later hand tinted. Although the hand-tinted images were often very effective representations of natural colors, photographers and scientists continued to be obsessed with the idea of making a fixed, realistic, color image directly from light. However, the black-and-white photograph did not come before the color photograph because it was imagined first. In their quest to produce relatively permanent color images, inventors simply discovered the black-and-white technology first.

To speak of black-and-white images in the nineteenth century is not entirely accurate. Many daguerreotypes, the first widely marketed "black-

and-white" photographic images, were actually quite colorful; however, they were monochromatic. Many daguerreotypes were actually mauve or brown. Thus, photographers could make "color" images in the mid-nineteenth century, but they could not make multicolored images, and they could not represent "real" colors directly from light.

When color photography finally became commercially available in the early decades of the twentieth century, it was met with widespread enthusiasm by many photographers, but not by a small group who felt the need to reject color photography definitively. Paradoxically, when color photography became easily available, some photographers began to promote black-and-white photography as never before. At the turn of the century, many photographers began to resent photography's status as an "objective," almost scientific endeavor. These photographers saw themselves as artists, not simply technicians. They saw their photographs as pieces of art, not simply as "documents." But in order to demonstrate their own creativity, these artists had to prove that nature itself was not doing all of their creating. They had to show that their works were not "real," but instead, the masterpieces of creative eyes and hands. They did everything possible to distance their images from reality. They chose black-and-white images over color images because it made their photographs seem at least one step removed from reality.

These self-proclaimed art photographers in the early decades of the twentieth century not only had to distance themselves from nature and science, but also from amateurs. When George Eastman marketed his first portable camera in the early twentieth century, it created a middle-class amateur photography boom. The snapshot was born, and photography became a tourist's primary occupation in foreign lands. One of Eastman's slogans— "You push the button, we do the rest"—made photography seem like a particular technical skill and certainly no particular artistic talent. Art photographers had to demonstrate that they were doing more than just pushing buttons. They had to distinguish their photographs from snapshots, in order to reveal the "deeper" meaning of their works. Many art photographers modeled their images after famous paintings. They created genre scenes and chose classic figures for their subjects. Art photographers took pictures of "Romeo and Juliet" on the cliffs, not pictures of May and Bill at the beach. They represented anguish, beauty, and joy; they did not document birthday parties, anniversaries, and weddings. Art photographers in the early twentieth century formulated their work as removed from reality and certainly as removed from "ordinary" reality.

8. Based on the author's description in the passage, the early inventors of photography might be called:

A. impatient.
B. imaginative.
C. creative.
D. persistent.

9. If an early twentieth-century art photographer were to walk into a late twentieth-century art gallery, which of the following pieces would he or she accept as art?

A. Hologram
B. Sculpture
C. Garden
D. Television

10. Based on the information given in the passage, one would surmise that early twentieth-century art photographers would have liked most to photograph:

A. their parents.
B. the President.
C. miners.
D. painters.

11. At some level, the author of the passage probably thinks that early art photographers were:

A. creative geniuses.
B. masters of technique.
C. clever capitalists.
D. insecure self-promoters.

12. In the early twentieth century, art was to reality as:

A. poetry is to prose.
B. books are to manuscripts.
C. radio is to television.
D. fiction is to nonfiction.

13. The passage implies that contemporary art photographers working with color photography are:

A. realistic.
B. clever.
C. practical.
D. unimaginative.

14. Documentary photography was developed in the same years that art photography was being distinguished from other types of photography. Because documentary photographers sought to show facts, they had to:

I. demonstrate their creative powers.
II. demonstrate their technical powers.
III. distance themselves from art.

A. I and II only
B. II and III only
C. I and III only
D. III only

15. Early inventors of photography were obsessed with the idea of making color photographs because color photographs were seen as:

A. realistic.
B. beautiful.
C. normal.
D. difficult.

Passage III (Questions 16–21)

Impressionism was given its name by a journalist of Charivari in 1874, who, in part, reacted to a painting of Monet titled, *Impression: Sunrise, 1872.* The origins of the impressionistic movement actually dated back to the mid-1860s, when Manet, Sisley, Bazille, and Monet began moving in a similar stylistic direction. This style emphasized the use of light, shadows, the atmosphere, and an emphasis on color with a relative independence of form. By the 1880s, many Parisian painters adopted the new impressionistic style. However, one of these painters, Toulouse–Lautrec, took impressionistic elements and applied them in original and interesting ways.

Henri de Toulouse–Lautrec was one of the most unique Parisian impressionist artists of the late nineteenth century. His artistic activity and personal destiny were as closely intertwined as other great artists of the time, such as Gauguin and Van Gogh. He was descended from an aristocratic family, namely the Counts of Toulouse. Although his father was healthy and an avid sportsman, Henri was an achondroplastic dwarf who could barely walk unaided. Henri's handicap was serious and played a major role in directing the course of his life and flavor of his art.

Toulouse–Lautrec was unable to blend into French society because of the stigmata of his deformity and his inability to accept rejection. Unable to lead the normal life of men in his aristocratic class, he soon withdrew from mainstream society and settled in Montmartre. During frequent trips to Paris, Toulouse–Lautrec would spend large amounts of time in cabarets. In this world of debauch and easy pleasure, he felt at ease as he did nowhere else. His acceptance in the evening establishments empowered him. With a keen sense of observation, Toulouse–Lautrec created dramatic, energetic, and passionate art with nightlife as his frequent subject matter.

There is no question that Toulouse–Lautrec was a bitter man, angered by his deformity, short stature, poor health, and helplessness to change his physical self. His bitterness is evident in his art, as the way he represented movement. The drawing is sharp and astringent, with an element of caricature. The coloring is aggressive, the subject matter frequently bizarre. He had an indifference to landscape but focused on artificial lighting and lines. Favorite subject matter included dancers, dance halls, circuses, women dressing, and female personalities.

In general, Toulouse–Lautrec's lithographs are as fine as his paintings and include some of his most authoritative work. Form is always subordinate to the expressive vitality of the outline. Some features of his human subjects are exaggerated for effect. Colors are concentrated and applied in large, flat areas, with unusual and striking harmonies. The use of color, dynamic drawing techniques, and a unique subject matter are what separate Toulouse–Lautrec from his contemporaries. In everything he did as an artist, Toulouse–Lautrec was an original, bold to the point of audacity.

The long-term effect of Toulouse–Lautrec still is felt today. His work had a significant influence on the development of modern art. Toulouse–Lautrec's style helped challenge official doctrines and encouraged painters to work to find a personal voice. With his better known, orthodox impressionist colleagues, Toulouse–Lautrec spoke of conveying movement and light in his paintings. In addition, the cultural aspect of the Parisian nightlife is forever recorded in the artist's posters of the Moulin Rouge and his paintings of famous personalities of the day, such as La Goulue, Jane Avril, and Valentin-le-Desosse.

16. According to the author, Toulouse–Lautrec's underlying impression of the world he lived in would be described as:

A. angry.
B. bitter.
C. just.
D. supportive.

17. Which of the following elements are important components of Toulouse–Lautrec's work?

I. Lines
II. Color
III. Contrast

A. I and II only
B. II and III only
C. I and III only
D. I, II, and III

18. The passage asserts that Toulouse–Lautrec felt comfortable in cabarets because:

A. he was an artist.
B. he was insecure in society.
C. he supported nightlife activities.
D. he was accepted there.

19. Impressionism differed from other art stylistic forms because:

A. impressionism stressed form and color more than style.
B. other artistic forms used light and shadows more than impressionism.
C. impressionism emphasized color with a relative independence of form.
D. other artistic forms ignore light, shadows, and the atmosphere.

20. Based on the description given in the passage, which term best describes Toulouse–Lautrec's artistic attitude?

A. Impudent
B. Arrogant
C. Flat
D. Aristocratic

21. The passage describes Toulouse–Lautrec's painting style as containing elements described as:

A. exaggeration and parody.
B. subtlety and nuances.
C. analysis and introspection.
D. bland and predictable.

Passage IV (Questions 22–28)

With all the advances we have made, we still have not come very far. Meteorologists have some of the most sophisticated machinery and data collection systems available, yet many of the complexities of Mother Nature still elude them. El Niño, the periodic disruption of normal weather patterns in the Pacific Ocean, wreaks economic and environmental havoc on the neighboring countries whenever it occurs. Although it is probably the largest force influencing global weather patterns, scientists still do not understand how it works or its cause.

El Niño means "the child" in Spanish. The phenomenon was so named because South America usually suffers its effects around Christmas time. The most recent El Niño occurred in 1992–1993, and damage caused by fire, drought, and floods on five continents was estimated at nearly 9 billion dollars. In India, Australia, southern Africa, Central America, and Indonesia, drought devastated crops and livestock (leading to malnutrition and starvation), depleted water supplies, and resulted in bush fires that killed more people and destroyed property. On the west Gulf Coasts of the United States, parts of South America, Hawaii, and Tahiti, violent storms and flooding destroyed property and crops, killed people, and left thousands homeless. Throughout the Pacific, warming ocean currents decimated birds and marine life and threw the normal ecosystem into imbalance. This devastated the commercial fishing industry and all those who rely on fish for business and as an inexpensive source of protein.

In the normal weather pattern, a high-pressure system is located in the eastern Pacific, near the coasts of North and South America. A wet, low-pressure system is located in the western Pacific above Indonesia. This causes trade winds to blow from east to west, generating a westward ocean surface current. This current accumulates warm water in the western Pacific, while cooler, deeper water recedes in an eastward current. When this cooler water reaches the coasts, it wells up, bringing with it rich nutrients that sustain the food chain. The cycle is continued as the water is warmed at the surface and pushed westward again by the trade winds.

When El Niño strikes, the high-pressure system breaks up and the low-pressure system shifts eastward. This disrupts and reverses the flow of the normal trade winds, resulting in dramatic shifts in normal weather patterns. Theses winds force warm surface waters towards North and South America in what is termed a Kelvin wave. Because the normal cycling is disrupted, the food chain falters and collapses. Despite its destruction, however, eventually El Niño ends, and the world gradually returns to normal.

Although these general ocean and weather patterns seem consistent from one El Niño to the next, the effects on the surrounding continents are not. In 1987–1988, California experienced severe drought, but in 1992–1993, much of the state suffered torrential rains and flooding. Although scientists do not know what triggers El Niño, some believe the winter monsoon may be the precipitating event. However, El Niño is a very complex weather event, and there may not be a single cause. Scientists currently are researching the phenomenon, hoping to be able to better predict when this disrupter of global climates may strike. Yet, will this do us any good? Ultimately everything we do revolves around the weather. Even if we are able to predict El Niño, can we do anything to prevent its devastation? As with all of Mother Nature's riddles, only time will tell.

22. In the third paragraph, the author's reference to the "coasts" refers to:

- **A.** the west coasts of North and South America.
- **B.** the east coasts of the Indonesian islands.
- **C.** coasts of small islands in the Pacific, such as Hawaii and Tahiti.
- **D.** the Gulf Coast of the United States.

23. Based on the information in the passage, it is reasonable to assume that:

- **A.** the Kelvin wave is responsible for generating tidal waves.
- **B.** the effects of an El Niño episode can be predicted because the weather pattern producing it is consistent.
- **C.** the food chain collapses during an El Niño event because there is no upwelling of nutrient-rich cool water.
- **D.** Central America experienced both drought and flooding during the 1992–1993 El Niño (although different regions).

24. The author would most likely support which of the following future scientific pursuits?

A. Developing more sophisticated machinery for predicting El Niño events
B. Investigating how to predict El Niño events
C. Investigating how to bring nutrient-rich waters up to the surface
D. Tabulating damage to lives and property caused by El Niño events

25. According to the passage, an El Niño develops when:

A. nutrient-rich waters fail to reach the surface.
B. a Kelvin wave moves eastward.
C. trade winds shift and blow northward.
D. the high-pressure system in the eastern Pacific dissipates, and the low-pressure system in the western Pacific migrates eastward.

26. In the last paragraph, the author states that "everything we do revolves around the weather." "Everything" most likely refers to all of the following EXCEPT:

A. agriculture.
B. commercial fishing.
C. city planning.
D. the progress of science.

27. The passage suggests that westward surface currents may be caused by winds that travel:

I. from the east.
II. toward the west.
III. toward the east.

A. I and III only
B. III only
C. I and II only
D. I, II, and III

28. According to the passage, the continental effects of El Niño are best described as:

A. serious.
B. expected.
C. difficult to define.
D. inconsistent.

Passage V (Questions 29–35)

The idealist philosopher, Benedetto Croce, was known to speak of history as essentially spiritual activity. His spiritual writings were understood in a thoroughly humanistic sense, without any explicit or implicit religious overtones. For Croce, it is the spiritual activity of man and his activity as a strictly human, rather than animal, being that provides meaning within history.

In a philosophical discussion with a colleague, Croce once posed the question, "What is knowledge by concepts?" According to Croce, it is the knowledge of the relations of things, and things are intuitions. Concepts are not possible without intuitions, just as intuition is itself impossible without the matter of impressions. Intuitions are this river, this lake, this brook, this rain, this cup of water; the concept is water, not this or that appearance and particular example of water, but water in general, in whatever time or place it be realized—the material of infinite intuitions, but of one single constant concept. Intuitions are also the inner meaning that connects the facts.

But the concept, the universal, if it be no longer intuition in one respect, is intuition in another respect and cannot fail of being intuition. The man who thinks has impressions and emotions, insofar as he thinks. His impression and emotion will be not love or hate, not the passion of the man who is not philosopher, not hate or love for certain objects and individuals, but the effort of his thought itself, with the pain and the joy, the love and the hate joined to it. This effort cannot but assume an intuitive form, in becoming objective to the spirit. To speak is not to think logically, but to think logically is also to speak.

The idea that thought cannot exist without speech is a truth generally admitted. The negations of this thesis are all founded on equivocations and errors. The first of the equivocations is that of those who observe that one can likewise think with geometrical figures, algebraical numbers, ideographic signs, without any word; even pronounced silently and almost insensibly within one.

Some people point out that certain animals think and reason without speaking. Now as to how, if, and what animals think, whether they be rudimentary men like savages who refuse to be civilized rather than physiological machines, are questions that do not concern us here. Analogy with man, knowledge of the spirit, human psychology, the instrument of all our conjectures as to animal psychology, would constrain us on the contrary to suppose that if they think in any way, they also somehow speak.

Adapted from Benedetto Croce, *Art and Philosophy.* © 1929 by Benedetto Croce.

29. According to the passage, Croce's writings may be described as:

I. humanistic.
II. spiritual.
III. religious.

A. I only
B. I and II only
C. II and III only
D. I and III only

30. Croce believed that ideas and thoughts were inherently tied to:

A. equivocations and errors.
B. ideographic signs.
C. impressions.
D. speech.

31. What is the purpose of the fifth paragraph in this passage?

A. To present an argument against the thesis discussed in the fourth paragraph
B. To defend the counterpoint raised in the third paragraph
C. To analyze the point brought up in the second paragraph
D. To address the question posed in the first paragraph

32. Based on the passage, which interdependency is LEAST supported?

A. Concepts:intuitions
B. Intuitions:impressions
C. Emotions:concepts
D. Thought:speech

33. Which event is a likely influence on Croce's ideas?

A. Vietnam War
B. Post-World War II politics
C. Russian Revolution
D. Civil War

34. Based on the Crocean principles discussed in the passage, which quality would one require to fully appreciate a work of art?

A. Concepts
B. Speech
C. Analysis
D. Intuition

35. Which term best describes the attitude of the author?

A. Defensive
B. Offensive
C. Idealistic
D. Idiosyncratic

Passsage VI (Questions 36–42)

Man's mind is ever busy contemplating one thought or another. His nature and habits are as his thoughts are. The fortunate have feelings of philanthropy toward others. In actively pursuing philanthropy for the good of others, these people make good use of their time and feelings and, thus, grow from strength to strength. These people are always rich with spirituality and never bring themselves down by minding other people's business.

To ensure one's own spiritual growth, self-thought and self-criticism are necessary conditions. If man forgets his true self, he focuses on his body and becomes deeply involved in body consciousness. This, in turn, subjects him to vices and the uneasiness and sorrow that follow such influences. To overcome such difficult circumstances, he can be redeemed by means of soul consciousness and vicelessness, which ultimately lead to true peace and happiness.

Fault finding is the greatest obstacle to spiritual development. From the worldly point of view, no one has the right to take the law into his own hands. In the field of spirituality, this rule of life is more stringent. The world is a variety show, and everyone's proclivities differ from every other's. So, it is wrong to hate anyone simply because his views are different from yours. If we try to punish anyone, we shall be losing our own spiritual strength and shall also become liable to punishment in accordance with our chosen religious leader. Hence, the spiritual aspirant should not only avoid seeing faults in others, but marking his own faults, try to be rid of them.

The ways of man's mind are difficult to analyze and judge because of the intricate pattern along which the mind works. There are feelings and fluctuations of the mind, with which man has to respond to fulfill or satisfy them. But the conscious mind does not accept them, with the result that the inner mind searches out other means of fulfilling itself. He ascribes these feeling to others and, thus, gets only a factitious form of satisfaction. He comes to think that he is free of those feelings, while others are bound by them. Thus, he is busy thinking of the defects of others, by which his own depraved tendencies get more deeply rooted in him. No one can deny the truth that those defects that he sees in others are manifest in himself. The external world is but a mirror, a projection in which is reflected our soul in its truest colors. We can see in that mirror our real identity.

Adapted from P.B. Kumaris, *Fault Finding Leads to One's Own Downfall.* © 1995 by P.B. Kumaris.

36. The passage suggests that fault finding leads to:

A. an improvement of the situation.
B. unpredictable changes.
C. destructive changes.
D. analysis and change.

37. The author encourages those seeking spiritual development to:

I. analyze the faults of others.
II. overlook the faults of others.
III. look for their own faults.

A. I only
B. I and III only
C. II and III only
D. III only

38. According to the author, faults that are identified in others are:

A. found widespread.
B. found in the fault finder.
C. feelings and fluctuations.
D. severe and obvious.

39. The passage links punishment with:

A. religious awakening.
B. acceptance of others.
C. self-thought and self-criticism.
D. loss of spiritual strength.

40. The ideals of which religious group are clearly advocated by the author?

A. Christianity
B. Islam
C. Judaism
D. None of the above. The author does not advocate any particular religious ideals.

41. According to the author, overinvolvement in the physical body may lead to:

A. spiritual deterioration.
B. self-thought.
C. vices.
D. loss of the conscious mind.

42. Which behavior is most advocated by the passage?

A. Tolerance
B. Constructive criticism
C. Spiritual changes
D. Seeking true happiness

Passage VII (Questions 43–50)

The Pacific Ocean is home to a wide variety of fish. Although most of these spend their entire life at sea, salmon are unusual in that they are born in streams, travel to the ocean where they mature, then return to the streams to breed. The Pacific is home to seven species of salmon, all belonging to the genus *Oncorhynchus*. There is a great diversity of weight among the varieties of salmon species. In order from smallest to largest average weight, they are: *O. garvuscha* (the pink, 4 pounds), *O. nerka* (the sockeye, 6 pounds), *O. masou* (the cherry, 9 pounds), *O. keta* (the chum, 9 pounds), *O. kisutch* (the coho, 9 pounds), *O. mykiss* (the steelhead, 9 pounds), and *O. tshawytscha* (the chinook or king, 22 pounds).

The life cycle of salmon begins with very small fish called alevins that hatch from fertilized eggs. These little ones have large pouches on their bellies that contain enough food to nourish them for several weeks. Alevins develop into fry; fry begin the journey downstream. Along the way, they must combat pollution, predators, and obstacles, such as the logging industry and dams. When they reach the river mouth, the salmon are termed *smolts*, and it is these finger-sized fish that make the transition from fresh to sea water.

When at sea, a Pacific salmon can travel as much as 10,000 miles as it moves from coastal waters to the deeper ocean depths and back again. As it travels, it gorges itself on zooplankton and small fish. It needs to sustain its rapid growth and lay down stores of muscle and fat to live on when it returns to fresh water. If it manages to escape pollution and predators at sea, the adult salmon returns to the river it left many months before. When it reaches the river, it must again negotiate the hazards as it makes its journey upstream. It is ironic that as a salmon grows into a full-sized adult, its main predator is man.

One of the most remarkable aspects about salmon is that they return to spawn at the exact location where they themselves were born. No one understands how they accomplish this. When the female reaches this spot, she digs a nest while several males surround her and fight for breeding rights. When they are done, the female lays her eggs as the winning male simultaneously discharges sperm to fertilize the eggs. The female then covers the eggs and begins to build another nest. At the end of the process, both partners die. The only exception is the *O. mykiss,* which can survive the ordeal to spawn multiple times.

Despite its spectacularity, the salmon's life cycle is wasteful and risky. Only about 0.1 percent of the eggs laid survives to spawn, and with man's continued encroachment on the salmon's habitat, the fish is increasingly threatened. However, man is exploring several ways to help. Fish farming is becoming popular as a means of improving the number of fish available for human consumption and decreasing the drain on wild salmon. Fry are being helped along their journey by releasing water from dams. Smolts are carried in helicopters from hatcheries and released into the sea. Passageways are built so that fish can get around dams. Hopefully, these attempts will help to preserve these natural wonders of the Pacific Northwest.

43. The passage claims that:

A. the steelhead is the species of Pacific salmon that lives the longest.
B. fry eat small plankton-like organisms found in fresh water.
C. chum salmon are usually larger than coho salmon.
D. larger species, such as the steelhead and chinook, have a better chance of surviving the obstacles in their journey upstream.

44. Which of the following statements about Pacific salmon are true?

I. They have mechanisms to cope with life in both fresh and salt water.
II. Man has endangered them.
III. They are unique in being the only genus of fish to live in both fresh and salt water.

A. I only
B. II only
C. I and II only
D. I, II, and III

45. The passage implies that:

A. adult salmon do not feed in fresh water when they return to spawn.
B. males that lose the fight for breeding rights with a female die without fertilizing any eggs.
C. larger species of salmon travel farther in the ocean then do smaller species.
D. the male protects the nest after the female covers the eggs.

46. According to the passage, one can conclude that:

A. female salmon lay their eggs in quiet areas of streams because faster moving water might carry the eggs away.
B. the largest male usually wins the fight for breeding rights.
C. a greater percentage of eggs laid survived to the point of spawning before the advent of modern man.
D. the predators of fry and adult salmon are the same in rivers.

47. If it were discovered that salmon locate their birthplace by "sensing" the correct chemical and nutrient composition of the water, then it could be reasonably inferred that:

A. salmon may have a more sophisticated sense of smell than humans.
B. new water pollution might affect a salmon's ability to return "home."
C. damage to a salmon's olfactory (smell) receptors during the course of its lifetime might cause it to return to the wrong location.
D. other fish likely have a similar mechanism they use to locate food sources.

48. The central thrust of this passage is that:

A. the Pacific salmon are endangered species.
B. man is becoming more aware of his impact on the environment.
C. salmon face may hazards because of the nature of their life cycle.
D. salmon are losing the battle with man.

49. According to the passage, the total number of salmon species is:

A. five.
B. seven.
C. nine.
D. not given.

50. Which fish would best survive in open sea environments?

A. Smolts
B. Fry
C. Alevins
D. Frawns

Passage VIII (Questions 51–58)

On October 12, 1992, Americans on both the northern and southern continents acknowledged the 500th anniversary of the day Christopher Columbus landed on the shores of what he thought were the Indies. Columbus' accidental "discovery" of new lands and peoples forever changed the course of world history. The way in which this event was remembered is the topic of a heated political debate that continues today.

Consider the famous phrase, "In 1492, Columbus sailed the ocean blue." That was all most people knew about Christopher Columbus until the recent proliferation of books, movies, and political demonstrations centered around the 1992 commemoration. While many are creating publications and films simply to capitalize on this major media event, others are attempting to reeducate people about the events of 500 years ago and the legacy of consequences stemming from those events. Still others are protesting a genocide.

According to Susan Shown Harjo, president and director of the Morning Star Foundation in Washington, DC, "We have no reason to celebrate an invasion." Harjo's foundation is sponsoring the 1992 Alliance, a group formed as part of an indigenous people's response to the Columbus Quincentenary. In an interview with Barbara Miner for Rethinking Schools, Harjo said the Alliance will focus its October 12 celebration this year on survival, the remarkable survival of Native Americans in the face of 500 years of oppression. According to Harjo, Native Americans will look toward the future, at the hope of the next 500 years this October 12.

Although this year a tremendous amount of energy is being focused on Columbus Day itself as a day some will celebrate and others will protest, many feel the bank holiday is not the only thing associated with Columbus that needs to be questioned. According to cultural critics such as Bill Bigelow, most of the children's books about Columbus and his adventures are based on and serve to reinforce white western racism. Many of the books focus on Columbus as a brave sailor and a great hero who "discovered" unpopulated lands or who brought Christianity and civilization to "savages." None of the books tell of Columbus' obsessive search for gold or the punishments he inflicted on indigenous people when they could not bring him enough gold. When Columbus himself had to admit there simply was no gold on the land, he began to take the native people back to Spain to sell as slaves.

Although these shocking tales do not make appropriate material for children's picture books, Bigelow would like to see new stories told. According to Bigelow, the problem with these children's books is not only the way Columbus is represented, but also the way the Native Americans are represented. None of the books mention that Native Americans had their own religions and cultures before Columbus came or that the Native Americans were generous to the newcomers. Conversely, none of the books mention that the Native Americans were brave resistance fighters. In short, none of the books narrate the events of Native Americans' point of view. The story of Columbus is always told as a conqueror's tale, from the conqueror's point of view.

October 12, 1992, offered us an opportunity to reflect on and reinterpret our mixed cultural history.

Adapted from Jonathan Majino, *The Columbus Commemoration Revisited.* © 1995 by Scholastic Press.

51. According to several viewpoints voiced in the passage, one might imagine changing Columbus Day to:

I. Native American Survival Day.
II. Native American Resistance Day.
III. Cultural Cooperation Day.

A. I and III only
B. I only
C. I and II only
D. I, II, and III

52. Columbus is often called a hero. He might also be called a:

A. tyrant.
B. detective.
C. historian.
D. diplomat.

53. The difference between "discovery" and "invasion" is:

A. historical.
B. perspective.
C. regional.
D. progressive.

54. Bill Bigelow would like to see more children's books about:

A. slavery.
B. brutality.
C. Native Americans.
D. gold.

55. According to the passage, Columbus' "discovery" might also be called:

A. a mistake.
B. history.
C. a plot.
D. a media event.

56. According to the passage, cultural producers see the October 12 Quincentenary variously as:

I. a marketing opportunity.
II. an opportunity to educate.
III. a political event to be ignored.

A. I, II, and III
B. I and III only
C. I only
D. I and II only

57. The author uses the phrase, "In 1492, Columbus sailed the ocean blue" to illustrate our relative:

A. racism.
B. childishness.
C. inferiority.
D. ignorance.

58. In the final paragraph of this passage, the author suggests that the reader should think about the Columbus Day celebration. Specifically, the author encourages the reader to:

A. plan a Columbus Day celebration.
B. ignore the Columbus Day celebration.
C. rethink the Columbus Day celebration.
D. write a children's book about the Columbus Day celebration.

Passage IX (Questions 59–65)

With the current politics of the antismoking crusade in mind, there might be a time in the future when a smoker could be arrested for smoking in public. The charge: endangering the lives of others or attempted murder. Does this sound far fetched? Perhaps, but with the Environmental Protection Agency's (EPA) recent report, described by Geoffrey Cowley in *Newsweek,* it is not unimaginable.

According to their latest investigation of respiratory health and what is called "passive smoking," inhaling the smoke exhaled by others (second-hand smoke) may be almost as lethal as first-hand smoke. In its still unofficial report, the EPA called ETS (environmental tobacco smoke) a "known human carcinogen." If this were to become an official assessment, ETS would be added to a long list of carcinogenic poisons that includes such deadly substances as arsenic and asbestos. If this were the case, smoking would probably be banned from all workplaces in the country.

Approximately two dozen cities and towns in the United States today have banned smoking in workplaces and restaurants. A few cities even have smoke-free bars and prisons, sites once considered smokers' havens. Although the number of smoke-free cities is still very small, many believe this may become a national trend. Just 2 years ago, there were only three smoke-free cities in the United States. Advocates of such measures claim that simply separating smokers from nonsmokers in the same room is not enough to protect nonsmokers from the harmful effects of ETS. ETS is not merely an annoyance, they claim, but a potentially life-threatening infringement on human health rights. Even if smoking and nonsmoking rooms were sealed off from one another and did not share the same air, workers at any establishment would be subject to the harmful effects of ETS.

According to the new EPA report, ETS might lead to 3000 lung cancer deaths each year. The report also attributes hundreds of thousands of infant respiratory infections each year to ETS, particularly smoke exhaled by parents. The findings also conclude that ETS starts thousands of new cases of asthma in young children each year and makes asthma worse for those children who already have it. The new EPA findings strengthen the claims of their earlier 1990 report and echo similar national research reports made as early as 1986. The EPA estimates that people who work or live with smokers have a 20%–30% higher risk of acquiring lung cancer than those who work and live only with nonsmokers. Although the EPA's investigation primarily focused on lung damage caused by ETS, many other researchers also claim that ETS increases heart disease in nonsmokers. The American Heart Association may begin its own research into this aspect of ETS.

The tobacco industry, a financially powerful political lobbyist, has been greatly disturbed by the results of the EPA research and is accusing them of biased studies. According to the Tobacco Institute, children are exposed to toxins of many different kinds, and respiratory problems cannot be traced definitively to exhaled tobacco smoke. The tobacco industry will undoubtedly fight to have the EPA's findings modified.

59. According to the passage, the Tobacco Institute:

- **A.** denies that environmental tobacco smoke (ETS) causes respiratory problems in children.
- **B.** denies that tobacco smoke may be toxic.
- **C.** tries to deflect attention away from the dangers of ETS.
- **D.** lies about ETS.

60. Some people claim that separating smokers from nonsmokers in the same room does not protect nonsmokers from environmental tobacco smoke (ETS) because:

- **A.** people occasionally smoke in the nonsmoking section.
- **B.** waiters move from one section to another.
- **C.** nonsmoking sections are too small.
- **D.** air circulates around a room.

61. One can infer from the passage that the Tobacco Institute's primary concern is:

- **A.** environmental.
- **B.** educational.
- **C.** political.
- **D.** self-interest.

62. If environmental tobacco smoke (ETS) were added to the list of official carcinogens, which ETS-related problem would be expected to develop and increase?

A. Lawsuits
B. Death threats
C. Asthma cases
D. Respiratory illnesses

63. If the Environmental Protection Agency's (EPA's) findings are correct, it is not unimaginable that parents who smoke near children might one day be accused of:

A. child abuse.
B. ignorance.
C. incompetence.
D. insanity.

64. The first paragraph of this passage is meant to:

A. annoy the reader.
B. offend the reader.
C. educate the reader.
D. surprise the reader.

65. Many health insurance agencies now charge smokers higher rates than nonsmokers. Based on information given in the passage, which other groups would be expected to also be charged with higher rates?

I. Children of smokers
II. Spouses of smokers
III. Bartenders

A. I and II only
B. I and III only
C. I, II, and III
D. I only

Solutions to Verbal Reasoning Practice Test 1

PASSAGE I

1. **D** The second paragraph of the passage emphasizes the weaknesses of the Tsar's army. The paragraph states that the army could only function as a coalition in the European arena. The passage does not indicate whether or not the army was a tested, predictable force. Choices A, B, and C are incorrect because they imply that the Tsar's army was either strong or tested. Choice D is best based on the negative description of the army given in the second paragraph.
2. **D** Start by finding the paragraph that uses the term *human locusts.* The third paragraph describes the Tsarist army failing at battle. The generals punished the peaceful population. People, most likely peasants, were driven off their land and pushed out of their homes. The final sentence of the paragraph summarizes the atrocity; the external rout (army losses by the enemy) was completed with an internal one (mistreatment and crimes against peasants).
3. **A** The author emphasizes in the last several sentences of the second paragraph that there were major class distinctions among Tsarist society. These class distinctions were important in determining one's role in Tsarist society. Thus, choice A is clearly supported by the passage. Choice B is partly a true statement. However, it is not as easily supported as choice A. Although some bourgeoisie may have been responsible for the injustices committed against peasants, this statement is too broad and encompassing. Outside of the army, there is no direct mention of mistreatment associated with social class. Choices C and D are not supported by the passage.
4. **C** This author is critical of Tsarist Russia. The criticism includes Russia's ambitions, the Tsarist army, and the Russian War Minister. Although the passage does provide some description, it is clearly partial. The passage provides very little unbiased analysis and significant censure.
5. **D** The fourth paragraph of the passage describes the reaction of the War Minister to early battle losses. The failure of the Tsarist army to deal with modern warfare was admitted by the War Minister in the first few sentences of this paragraph. The use of human mobilizations (poor fighters/soldiers) to overwhelm the enemy with bodies was described as an unforgivable battle strategy. This unsuccessful strategy led to over 5 million casualties.
6. **A** The passage clearly shows class distinction. The example given was within the army. The peasants were foot soldiers, and the commanders were the ruling classes and bourgeoisie. Choice B is incorrect because equality was never discussed or described in the passage. Economic depression may be inferred to some degree; however, it is not as easily supported as choice A. Choice D is not supported by the passage.

7. **D** The author of the passage does not say that Russian involvement in the war could have been prevented. On the contrary, the author states that "Russia could not help participating in the scramble." Thus, choice A is incorrect. Choice B is not supported because the passage does not indicate whether or not Russia was provoked into becoming involved in the war. In addition, the passage does not discuss political ramifications of battle losses, so eliminate choice C.

PASSAGE II

8. **D** Choices B and C are synonymous and are not supported by the passage; the author does not stress the creativity of the inventors. Choice A is incorrect because the passage emphasizes the time required to develop a color photographic process. "Persistent" best describes the early inventors of photography.
9. **A** This is a difficult inference question. Look for a place in the passage that discusses how early twentieth-century art photographers thought of their work. Paragraph three indicates that the photographers did everything possible to distance their images from reality. In other words, they sought to distance art from "real" representations. When considering answers, look for the choice that is most distant from reality. Of the choices given, holograms are the most distant from reality.
10. **D** The fourth paragraph covers this topic in some detail. The author clearly states that art photographers modeled their images after famous paintings. It is also implied that early twentieth-century art photographers did not want to make family snapshots or documentary images (of the President or miners).
11. **D** See paragraphs three and four. The general tone of these paragraphs and the way the author uses quotation marks around key words are almost sarcastic. There is a subtle, negative attitude expressed by the author. Note that many of the quoted phrases are promotional words or phrases; this best fits choice D.
12. **D** Note that choices A and B both contain elements that are closely related to each other. Poetry is prose and books are often manuscripts at one time. Choice C describes two media that also are related. Radio is a communication medium, as is television. However, choice D describes opposites. Fiction is the opposite of nonfiction. Paragraph three suggests that in the early twentieth century, art was conceived of as different from realistic or "objective" documentation. This means that the most divergent choice is likely the best (choice D).
13. **B** Paragraph five discusses contemporary art photographers. This new work is not "realistic" in the ways that we are generally accustomed. The author uses the term *alternative realities* to describe this work. Thus, eliminate choice A. Choices C and D are not supported because the author does not discuss practicality and imagination. The author does indirectly imply that the art photographers are clever.

14. **B** By inverting the claims of the art photographers, we can infer the claims documentary photographers might have made. Statement I would most likely resemble a statement an art photographer would make. Statements II and III would most likely be made by a documentary photographer. Thus, choice B is best.
15. **A** Paragraph one states that photographers were obsessed with creating a realistic, fixed color image. The process of hand tinting black-and-white images to portray realistic colors is also presented. These provide evidence that early inventors of color photography were obsessed because color photographs were realistic.

PASSAGE III

16. **B** The fourth paragraph indicates that Toulouse–Lautrec was a bitter man who was angered by his deformed body. This bitterness is stated to have affected his art and his attitude. There is no support of choices A, C, or D in the passage.
17. **A** The importance of outline and drawing techniques is discussed in the passage and support statement I. Statement II is supported throughout the passage, particularly in the fourth and fifth paragraphs. Statement III is not discussed in the passage. Thus, choice A (I and II) is best.
18. **D** The passage emphasizes Toulouse–Lautrec's deformity and the effects it had on him. The third paragraph explains that Toulouse–Lautrec chose to spend time in places that accepted him, such as cabarets. The other choices are not supported by the passage.
19. **C** To answer this question, note that a general discussion of impressionism is given in the first paragraph. The third sentence of the first paragraph indicates that impressionism placed emphasis on color with a relative independence of form. This directly supports choice C.
20. **A** If you do not know what impudent means, use the process of elimination to evaluate the other answer choices first. Choice B is incorrect because Toulouse–Lautrec's artistic attitude is not arrogant. Toulouse–Lautrec's attitude is best described as bold and flashy. Choice C can be eliminated because Toulouse–Lautrec's attitude is anything but flat. The passage does not support the artist's attitude as aristocratic. Choice D may also be eliminated. Although he descended from an aristocratic family, Toulouse–Lautrec's artistic attitude was not mainstream or aristocratic. Toulouse–Lautrec was audacious and brazen (impudent).
21. **A** The fifth paragraph describes Toulouse–Lautrec's work. It is discussed in terms of colors, unusual and striking harmonies, and exaggeration of features in human subject pieces. The exaggeration of human features (e.g., large noses) suggests parody. Choices B and D are far from accurate descriptions of Toulouse–Lautrec's painting style. The artist was bold and painted with little subtlety. He was not bland and predictable. In addition, the passage does not indicate that his work contained introspection and analysis.

PASSAGE IV

22. **A** The third paragraph overviews the trade wind direction and its effect on producing an ocean current. This paragraph supports that the cooler ocean current moves eastward, toward the west coasts of North and South America.

23. **C** The third paragraph states that the cool, upwelling water brings up the nutrients that sustain the food chain. When El Niño occurs, this cycle is disrupted, and the food chain collapses. Choice A is incorrect because Kelvin waves are not mentioned as responsible for tidal waves. Choice B is false. The passage indicates that El Niño is periodic, but episodes are not predictable and consistent. Choice D is incorrect because the drought and flooding discussed took place in California.

24. **B** Look for evidence in the passage to support one of the choices. In the last paragraph, the author says that scientists are still working to learn how to predict El Niños. This lends support to choice B, which is the best answer. The other investigations are not mentioned.

25. **D** This question may be easily answered from information drawn directly from the passage. The first few sentences of paragraph four support choice D. Choices A, B, and C are there to distract you. Notice that these choices use terminology from the fourth paragraph and require that you systematically evaluate them by the process of elimination.

26. **D** El Niño is destructive because it disrupts or destroys activities that are dependent on the weather or ocean environment. Choices A, B, and C all meet this description. For example, if an area is repeatedly experiencing flooding from El Niño events, it would not be wise to build a city in that area. Choice D is the correct response to this question, as it is the choice that is least dependent on the weather.

27. **C** This question tests to see if you can correctly identify the current and wind relationships described in the passage. First, note that these relationships are mentioned in paragraph three. Second, evaluate each statement to see which is correct. Statements I and II are correct based on the description given in paragraph three. Statement III is not supported by the passage. Thus, choice C is best.

28. **D** Carefully evaluate each choice to see which fits the tone and message of the passage best. Choice A may be a true statement, but it is quite vague. What does serious mean? Damaging or not comical? Choice B is incorrect based on the element of El Niño unpredictability described in the passage. Choice C is ambiguous; the continental effects of El Niño are not difficult to define. Effects are measurable. Choice D most accurately describes the continental effects of El Niño. The passage goes into much detail outlining the variability and inconsistencies of El Niño.

PASSAGE V

29. **B** This question asks general information about Croce's writings. This is discussed in the first paragraph. Make a mental map of the passage as you read to help recall what information is contained where. Paragraph one indicates that Croce's writings are spiritual and human oriented (statements I and II). The passage does not support any particular religious theme to Croce's writings (statement III). Thus, B (I and II only) is correct.

30. **D** The first sentence of the fourth paragraph states that thought cannot exist without speech. This ties together thoughts and speech. Equivocations and errors are discussed in the fourth paragraph but not clearly tied to thoughts. Impressions are tied to intuitions in the third paragraph. The term *idolgraphic signs* is mentioned in the fourth paragraph, but it does not relate to the question asked.

31. **A** Use the process of elimination to answer this question. Carefully look at the fifth paragraph, and review what is covered topically. Note that this paragraph relates to speech. An argument is made that points out that animals cannot speak, yet they reason and think. This is a contradiction to the fourth paragraph, which emphasizes that thought cannot exist without speech. Thus, choice A is a correct statement. The fifth paragraph presents an argument against the thesis discussed in the fourth paragraph. Now quickly evaluate the other choices. Choice B is not a true statement; the third paragraph does not appear to present a counterpoint. Choice C is false because the second paragraph defines the relationships among concepts, intuitions, and impressions; it has nothing to do with speech. Choice D is false because the first paragraph does not pose a question. Choice A is best by the process of elimination.

32. **C** Choices A and B are supported by the relationships defined in paragraph two. Choice D is supported by the relationship given in paragraph four. Only emotions to concepts (choice C) are not interrelated in the passage.

33. **C** As discussed in Chapter 4, citations that follow passages contain important clues. In this passage, the citation shows that the passage was adapted from writings published in 1929. This places a distinct timeline on the piece. Choices A and B can be eliminated because they are historical events that occurred years after 1929. Now choose between choices C and D. Based on the tone and content of the passage, which is a more reasonable influence? First, Croce likely lived during the period of the Russian Revolution (1917) and not during the period of the Civil War (1860s). Second, the piece has an almost Marxist flavor to it. Both of these factors would favor choice C.

34. **D** This difficult question requires inference. Use the process of elimination to select the most plausible answer. Concepts are described in paragraph two as the knowledge of the relations of things. This would not relate to appreciating a work of art. Speech is related to thought in the

fourth paragraph, but speech would not apply to art appreciation easily. Analysis is not discussed in the passage. Intuition is described as "things" in the second paragraph. Intuition is also described as the inner meaning that connects the facts. Art has both a physical form and an inner meaning to the person who appreciates it. Thus, choice D appears to best describe a Crocean quality required for art appreciation.

35. **C** The passage overviews some of the ideas of a philosopher. The author does not defend a particular viewpoint. Similarly, the author does not go on the offensive attacking another viewpoint. The passage demonstrates no idiosyncrasies. The author is idealistic and visionary.

PASSAGE VI

36. **C** The take-home message of this passage is given in the citation at the end of the passage. The citation states that faultfinding leads to one's own downfall. This suggests that faultfinding is destructive. This best supports choice C.

37. **C** This author writes with a far-eastern, religious style. In paragraph three, he encourages the reader to overlook the faults of others (statement II) and to look inward to find one's own faults (statement III). The author does not encourage those seeking spiritual development to analyze the faults of others. Thus, statements II and III are true, and choice C is best.

38. **B** Evaluate each choice carefully, and eliminate choices lacking support from the passage. In the second half of the fourth paragraph, the author implies that a person should look inward to discover that defects (faults) that are noted within others are manifest in self. This directly supports choice B. The author does not say that faults are widespread, although to some degree, this may be implied. However, choice B is better supported in the passage than choice A. Choices C and D lack any support from the passage.

39. **D** Hopefully, you identified "punishment" as a key word in the passage. Go back to the passage quickly and find where this word was used. Note its use in the third paragraph. The author links the loss of spiritual strength with religious punishment. Choices A, B, and C are not linked with "punishment" in the passage.

40. **D** This is a tricky inference question. You are asked to draw from the passage any religious overtones and decide if a religious faith is clearly supported. Because the author does not discuss any direct religious group in the passage, you can make your decision only based on implications. The passage is very spiritual, but the author does not appear to direct the reader toward any particular faith. As a matter of fact, at the end of the third paragraph, the author uses the phrase "our own chosen religious leader." Even though the passage carries some elements of far-eastern religious philosophy, there is not enough evidence to clearly support the advocations of any faith.

41. **C** The second paragraph of the passage discusses the risk of forgetting true self. Overinvolvement in body consciousness is tied to vices and sorrow in the second and third sentences of this paragraph. This strongly supports choice C. Choice A, spiritual deterioration, may occur with overinvolvement in the physical body, but this is not as clearly stated or supported as choice C. Choice B, self-thought, is mentioned in the first sentence of the second paragraph, but this is not given as a result of physical body overinvolvement. Choice D is not discussed or supported in the passage.

42. **A** This question indirectly asks you to draw the main idea from the passage. Think about what the author is trying to convey in the passage. The citation gives you a strong clue. The author is encouraging the reader to be less critical of others. He advocates one's own spiritual growth, and he deplores faultfinding. The author appears to be a live-and-let-live person. Carefully evaluate each choice. Choice A is supported by the passage. The tolerance of others is clearly a behavior that the author advocates. Choice B is incorrect. The passage does not encourage criticism of any kind even if it is constructive. Choices C and D are not as good as choice A. Although spiritual changes and seeking true happiness are likely things that the author supports, the passage does not focus on these behaviors.

PASSAGE VII

43. **A** This is a good example of an expository passage. The passage is full of information giving details about the Pacific salmon. To answer this question specifically, you must evaluate the accuracy of each statement given as an answer choice. Start with choice A. Notice that details are given for salmon by species name. Find the paragraph in the passage that gives the species name for steelhead salmon. Paragraph one gives the species name for steelhead salmon as *Oncorhynchus mykiss*. Paragraph four states that *O. mykiss* does not die after the initial spawning but can survive to spawn several times. This suggests that steelhead salmon live the longest of the species mentioned. The other choices are not supported by the passage.

44. **C** The passage supports statements I and II. Note that statement III is a restrictive statement. In general, such restrictive statements are rarely true in the MCAT Verbal Reasoning section. To negate such statements, all you have to do is find one exception to the statement or find that such a restriction is not supported by the passage. In this case, the passage does not state that Pacific salmon are the only genus to live in both fresh and salt water. Thus, choice C (statements I and II) is best.

45. **A** This is an inference question. Note that paragraph three mentions that salmon need to lay down stores of muscle and fat to sustain themselves when they return to fresh water. This implies that salmon do not feed in fresh water and supports choice A. Choices B and D are not supported. The fourth paragraph does discuss the role of male

salmon in breeding, but only as fertilizer of the eggs. Choice C is not discussed in the passage.

46. **C** When a question asks you to arrive at a conclusion, look for a theme that is carried in two or more paragraphs. Frequently, the author will ask you about that theme. Notice that the passage mentions in several places that man is negatively affecting the salmon's habitat and breeding. The last paragraph of the passage states that man is increasingly threatening the salmon and, thus, further decreasing the percentage of eggs laid that survive to the point of spawning. This supports choice C. The other choices are either false statements or unsupported statements.

47. **B** Work through the choices to see which is most reasonable based on information given in the passage. Answer choices A and C involve the sense of smell. The information contained in the question does not imply that "sensing" is equivalent to smell. One would incorrectly have to equate "sensing" and "smell" to choose choice A or C. Choice D is not supported by the passage because only salmon are discussed. Choice B is the best choice, as water pollution might alter the chemical and/or nutrient balance of the water and affect "sensing."

48. **C** This is a "main theme" question. Although the passage does discuss the negative effect that man is having on the salmon, the passage does not state or suggest that salmon are endangered or losing a "battle" with man. Thus, eliminate choices A and D. Choice B is incorrect because the passage does not discuss mankind's awareness of the environment. Choice C is best supported. The passage emphasizes the life cycle of the salmon and the hazards that they face at various stages in this cycle.

49. **D** This question tests if you overconclude or do not read for details. The passage gives seven species of Pacific salmon. The passage does not mention how many total salmon species there are. Be careful in apparently simplistic questions like this. The author would not have asked the question if it were so easy.

50. **A** The second paragraph of the passage provides all the information you need to answer this question. The passage indicates that alevins develop into fry; fry then begin the journey downstream (in fresh water). Fry are known as smolts when they reach the river mouth and enter the sea. Thus, B and C are incorrect. Choice D is a nonsensical term. Choice A is the best choice.

PASSAGE VIII

51. **C** Both statements I and II are supported by the passage. In the third paragraph, the author indicates that the Alliance focused its celebration on survival of Native Americans. In paragraph five, Native Americans are portrayed as brave resistance fighters. There is no mention of cultural cooperation in the passage. Thus, choice C (I and II) is best.

52. **A** The fourth paragraph of the passage portrays Columbus in a negative light. This paragraph dispels the image of Columbus as a brave sailor and hero and describes Columbus as a driven, tyrannical man. Choice B is not as good as choice A. Detective work is not directly discussed in the passage, although one could extrapolate Columbus' search for gold as some sort of detective work. Columbus is not discussed as a historian, so eliminate choice C. Choice D is not directly supported and carries more of a positive connotation; the fourth paragraph of the passage is certainly negative in tone.
53. **B** Look for places in the passage that use the words *discovery* and *invasion*. Note that these words are used in the third and fourth paragraphs. The word *discovery* is used in discussing Bill Bigelow's work and his challenges to the current teachings about Columbus. The word *invasion* is used in the third paragraph as a quotation from Susan Harjo and appears to have a negative connotation. These two words voice different positions or standpoints. Choice B (perspective) best describes the difference between these two words.
54. **C** Bigelow does not advocate telling children tales of brutality. Thus, choices A and B are unlikely. Choice D is not supported. Bigelow does not emphasize gold or other materialistic items. Choice C (Native Americans) is the topic about which Bigelow wants to educate children.
55. **A** The first paragraph describes Columbus' discovery of the new lands as "accidental." Choice A is the closest choice to accidental. Choices B, C, and D do not accurately describe the context of the "discovery" as used in the first paragraph.
56. **D** The passage describes the value and meaning of Columbus Day to various individuals and groups. Marketing (capitalistic ventures) is discussed in the second paragraph, making statement I true. The "reeducation" of people is discussed in the third sentence of the second paragraph. This lends support to statement II. Statement III is not supported by the passage.
57. **D** In the first sentence of the second paragraph, this phrase is used to point out how little most people knew about Columbus. This supports the use of the word *ignorance*. Choices A, B, and C can be eliminated because racism, childishness, and inferiority are not discussed in relation to this phrase in the second paragraph.
58. **C** The final question in this passage is probably the easiest. Use the process of elimination to evaluate each choice. The author does not encourage the reader to plan a Columbus Day celebration or to ignore Columbus Day. Furthermore, the author does not encourage the reader to write a book about Columbus Day. The intentions of the author are emphasized in the sixth paragraph; Columbus Day provides an opportunity to reflect upon our history.

PASSAGE IX

59. **C** The strategies of the Tobacco Institute are discussed in the fifth paragraph. The Tobacco Institute stresses the dangers of other kinds of toxins, not tobacco smoke. This supports choice C. Choice A is not clearly supported in the passage. The Tobacco Institute argues that toxins other than tobacco smoke may cause respiratory problems in children. Choice B is incorrect because the Tobacco Institute does not deny that tobacco smoke may be toxic. Choice D is false because there is no discussion or evidence given in the passage to support that the Tobacco Institute lies about environmental tobacco smoke (ETS).

60. **D** This topic is discussed in the third paragraph. It is implied that smokers and nonsmokers would not share the same air if they were in separate rooms. Conversely, it can be assumed that while seated in the same room, smokers and nonsmokers share the same air.

61. **D** See paragraph five. The Tobacco Institute is described as a financially powerful political lobbyer that will surely fight against the Environmental Protection Agency's (EPA's) findings. This supports the choice that the Tobacco Institute's motivation is self-interest. This is the best choice. Choice C is an accurate statement but not as descriptive or specific as choice D. The passage does not support that the Tobacco Institute's main concern is either environmental or educational.

62. **A** Health effects would not necessarily change because of this classification, but legal issues might. See paragraph two. If smoke is designated a carcinogen, smoking might be banned legally from public places. In addition, tobacco smoke could be considered a cancer-causing poison whose exposure places people at a health risk. This could lead to lawsuits and damage awards.

63. **A** Paragraph four discusses the Environmental Protection Agency (EPA) report and its findings. Paragraph one indicates that there may be a time in the future when a smoker could be held accountable for the effects of cigarette smoke on others. With the tone of the first paragraph in mind, it makes sense that parents who smoke near children might be damaging them physically (child abuse). Although ignorance might be exhibited by parents who smoke near children, the passage does not discuss this. Incompetence and insanity are neither discussed nor implied.

64. **D** You should note that the first paragraph in this passage is bold and immediately makes strong statements. What is the purpose of this writing style? Surprise. Notice that the author of the passage asks if the event described in the first two sentences of paragraph one seems far-fetched.

65. **C** See paragraphs three and four. Children and spouses of smokers are constantly exposed to environmental tobacco smoke (ETS). This supports statements I and II. Bartenders tend to work in smoke-filled rooms. This supports statement III. Thus, choice C (I, II, and III) is the best choice.

VERBAL REASONING PRACTICE TEST 2

Suggested Time: 85 minutes

Directions: There are nine reading passages in the Verbal Reasoning test. Each passage is followed by several questions. After reading a passage, select one best answer to each question. If you are not certain of an answer, eliminate the alternatives that you know to be incorrect, and then select an answer from the remaining alternatives.

Passage I (Questions 1–7)

Although many Americans assume that English is the official language of the United States, it is not. Nowhere in the United States Constitution is English privileged over other languages, and although a few subsequent federal laws require the use of English for special, limited purposes—traffic control, product labels, warnings, official notices, service on federal juries, and naturalization of immigrants—no law establishes English as the language of the land.

On the other hand, Americans often assume that all the world speaks English, or that it should; the image of the "ugly" American abroad hinges in part on this frequently thwarted linguistic expectation. They further assume that everyone in the United States speaks English, or should. Moreover, many English-speaking Americans tend to regard English not just as a language, but as an essential human trait. Consequently, nonanglophones may be regarded not simply as un-American, but as subhuman. To cite one egregious example, Daniel Shanahan reports that in 1904 a railroad president once told a congressional hearing on the mistreatment of immigrant workers, "These workers don't suffer—they don't even speak English."

Just as the American stereotype assumes monolingual competence in English, American legislatures, courts, and schools have always operated on the assumption that English is indeed the official language of public expression—that English is the normal vehicle of the government, courts, schools, and general business community in the United States. Although the legal record is generally silent or unclear on this matter, the assumption that English is or should be official occasionally has been voiced by political leaders and federal courts. For example, in 1923 the United States Supreme Court, in a decision protecting foreign language instruction in the schools, ventured the opinion that it was desirable for English to be the American national language (*Meyer v. Nebraska,* 262 US 390). As early as 1780, John Adams predicted the United States would be the vehicle for making its national language, English, the next world language "because the increasing population in America . . . will . . . force their language into general use, in spite of all the obstacles that may be thrown in the way." John Quincy Adams opposed the Louisiana Purchase because "it naturalizes foreign nations in a mass." In 1807, President Thomas Jefferson, who held similar fears that immigrants coming from absolute monarchies would be unable to adjust to American principles and would transmit their language to their children, proposed settling some 30,000 Americans—whom he assumed to be speakers of English—in the newly acquired Louisiana Territory to prevent that area from remaining French in language and law.

The motives for privileging English are often simply practical or patriotic; proponents of official English assume that a nation functions best if its citizens share a common language, although it is clear that there are no monolingual nation-states today and that, contrary to the myth of Babel, plurilingualism may always have been the basic human condition. In any case, supporters of official-language laws hope that imposing English by statute will accelerate its adoption among nonanglophones, though the furor over bilingual education and the generally disappointing experience with foreign language requirements in school curricula might suggest the futility of forcing anyone to learn a language.

Adapted from Dennis Baron, *The English-Only Question.* © 1990 by University Press.

1. Which of the following conclusions would best describe the central theme of the passage?

A. Efforts to establish a truly monolingual nation are relatively futile.
B. Attempts to establish English as the official language of the United States have a long and arduous history.
C. English has been acknowledged only recently as the official language of the United States.
D. Efforts at establishing English as the official language of the United States traditionally have been grounded in concerns about national identity.

2. Based on information in the passage, it is reasonable to assume that the author:

A. is in favor of efforts to privilege the use of English in the United States.
B. challenges efforts to privilege the use of English in the United States.
C. is relatively indifferent to efforts to privilege the use of English in the United States.
D. fears efforts to privilege the use of English in the United States.

3. According to the historical information provided by the author, which of the following statements best describes past political actions regarding language rights in America?

A. Politicians have made concerted efforts to deny immigrants the right to speak their native languages.
B. Legislation regarding language in the United States historically has been based on the xenophobia of politicians.
C. The historical acquisition of territory has been guided largely by concerns over language.
D. Efforts to naturalize foreign masses have been relatively indirect.

4. The passage assumes that non-English speakers present a threat to the United States based on:

A. their inability to communicate effectively with English speakers.
B. their insistence that foreign languages be taught in American schools.
C. their subhuman qualities.
D. their failure to assimilate effectively.

5. On the basis of the author's comments about the possibility of forcing individuals to learn a foreign language, which of the following statements seems most accurate?

A. Americans will always be averse to the establishment of anything but English as the official language.
B. The acquisition of a second language is always a complicated and difficult task.
C. Americans are far too idealistic to assume that legislating an official language is a viable and reasonable alternative to plurilingualism.
D. Americans generally are unreceptive to the learning of other languages.

6. Observations made by the author about the average American appear to suggest that most Americans:

A. regard English as the universal language.
B. assume that most non-Americans speak at least some English.
C. expect that non-Americans should at least make the effort to learn some English.
D. assume that non-English speakers should not be allowed the same rights as English speakers.

7. Based on information in the passage, it would seem reasonable to assume that:

A. plurilingualism is the most likely prospect for the United States.
B. efforts by supporters of official-language laws are likely to intensify.
C. the future of language legislation in the United States is relatively ambiguous.
D. efforts by supporters of official-language laws are likely to diminish.

Passage II (Questions 8–14)

There is little doubt that the celebration of Halloween in the United States has diminished dramatically over the last 10 years. Because of such things as the recklessness commonly associated with October 31, as well as growing fears for the safety of children, many Americans appear to have abandoned the day altogether. What was once a holiday eagerly anticipated by candy and party lovers alike has unfortunately become a target of derision. I say unfortunately because Americans appear to have forgotten the importance of Halloween and the fact that the "manageable" problems associated with it are far outweighed by its benefits. Louise Krasniewicz, an anthropologist, provides perhaps the best explanation of what I mean.

Krasniewicz has come out as an academic against concerted efforts to ban the celebration. Specifically, she cites the recent scrutiny by the Los Altos school board, which unsuccessfully tried to ban Halloween costumes under the guise that Halloween is a religious holiday. Other school boards have also tried to eliminate Halloween costumes as inappropriate and offensive.

However, she notes that this effort to ban costumes, for whatever reason, misses the whole point of this special day. Halloween is the one and only day of the year across the United States when it should be appropriate to turn the world on its head and do the outrageous, ridiculous, and insulting things that are not acceptable the rest of the year. We not only enjoy such days, we actually need them. It is during such rituals of role reversal and simulated lawlessness that we see just what will tear our world apart and how we can safely put it back together again.

On Halloween, the boundaries between good taste and bad, living and dead, fantasy and reality, and humans and nonhumans come tumbling down. In the Halloween world, nothing is as it seems and everything is called into question. The most basic categories by which we usually order our world collapse on Halloween and for one night the dead walk, beasts talk, inanimate objects come to life, and men and women are interchangeable.

When you join the Halloween masquerade, you contribute your own particular vision to creating a topsy-turvy world. Men can be Superman or Marilyn Monroe. A feminist can be a cheerleader, a scientist can consult a gypsy fortuneteller, and a pacifist can lust after General Patton. The gruesome or disgusting become objects of fun. The sacred is ridiculed. The rogue becomes admirable.

On Halloween, children, like adults, get to try out and therefore control unruly characters or attitudes that may frighten or intrigue them, and they seem to relish and understand the value of this. At any other time, such bizarre reversals or experiences might be terrifying and unbearable. On Halloween, they are embraced.

Throughout history and around the world, cultures have created ritual events during which people face those things that can make their society come apart at the seams. The most famous examples are Carnival in Brazil and Mardi Gras in the United

States. By highlighting the taboo and antisocial in an acceptable setting, people reaffirm the values of a society's "normal life."

Although Halloween originated in part as a harvest festival and pagan religious activity, we now emphasize the fantastical side, tailoring it to the fears we have about living in the present-day world. Yet Halloween also helps us to see that our society is goofy, crazy, fascinating, imaginative, contradictory, and ever-changing, and that it has the potential to be renewed.

Adapted from Louise Krasniewicz, *Halloween: Should We or Shouldn't We?* © 1997 by Louise Krasniewicz.

8. Based on the passage, Halloween has been abandoned in the United States largely because of its:

A. historical roots.
B. contemporary character.
C. psychological disadvantages.
D. anthropological consequences.

9. Which of the following statements best illustrates the connection made in the passage between Halloween and the fears of Americans?

A. The celebration of Halloween essentially is based on a misguided fear of the unknown and unfamiliar.
B. Our fear of Halloween essentially is based more in irrationality than rationality.
C. The relationship between fear and Halloween is essentially advantageous.
D. The most significant objection to Halloween in the United States is based on fears of complicating the separation of church and state.

10. Based on the more attractive "possibilities" engendered by Halloween as suggested in the passage, which of the following observations seems most accurate?

A. Standard social boundaries generally are weak and easily manipulated.
B. Standard social boundaries are too rigid and must be challenged periodically.
C. Standard social boundaries are dangerously vague and ambiguous.
D. Standard social boundaries are highly fluid.

11. The claim that Halloween allows us to "see just what will tear our world apart and how we can put it back together again" suggests that:

A. there are forces at work in American society that consistently threaten social order and stability.
B. simulated lawlessness can, in fact, prevent genuinely dangerous lawlessness.
C. fantasy and role reversal can help to maintain important social boundaries.
D. the distinction between the acceptable and the unacceptable is culturally relative.

12. Based on the logic of the passage, the celebration of Halloween best illustrates the underlying:

A. creativity of Americans.
B. anxiety of Americans.
C. depravity of Americans.
D. craziness of Americans.

13. According to the author, the trends in American social life that appear to be contributing to the condemnation of Halloween suggest:

A. a more widespread concern about crime and lawlessness in general.
B. a growth of conservatism in the United States.
C. a more widespread concern about maintaining order in schools.
D. a general frustration with the decline of religion in America.

14. The author's observation that the problems of Halloween are "manageable" most probably means that:

A. most Americans tend to observe Halloween in relatively peaceful terms.
B. the problems associated with Halloween are relatively nonthreatening.
C. we should be willing to accept the minor problems associated with Halloween, considering the relative advantages of the holiday.
D. all of the above.

Passage III (Questions 15–20)

Being trained and obtaining status as a new professional constitute only the beginning of a career. Subsequently, most scientists' professional careers are unproductive and unnoticed by most of society. They may be good teachers, advisers, citizens, and employees, but they are not productive scientists. Productive members of the scientific community are rare. Publication (frequently used to measure productivity) for a given group follows Lotka's "law of distribution," which states, in part, that 5% of the scientists will produce 50% of the literature in a field, whereas 50% will produce only 5% of the publications.

It is possible for a scientist to gain rewards as a member of either an organization, the scientific community, or both. A member of an organization joins committees, works to improve his institution and his own standing in it, and generally focuses his attention locally. A member of the scientific community spends most of his time on his professional associates.

Two facts of scientific life lead to individual tragedy. First, scientists "age"; most do not change their techniques or ideas after their PhD training has been completed. Second, new ideas or techniques develop with some regularity. In engineering, where skills are directly usable in technological processes, it can become painfully obvious rapidly when a person no longer has the skills to do a particular job. Engineers call this "technological obsolescence," and some effort has been made to provide retraining. Scientific obsolescence is less a matter of technology than of conceptual schemes. Scientists who simply fail to understand or accept changes in the way in which a field's conceptual scheme is being modified gradually become uninvolved in the current ideas of their disciplines. They may be excellent administrators, teachers, or deans, but they are no longer productive scientists.

Unemployment is particularly critical for scientists because of the knowledge obsolescence discussed previously. In many fast-growing areas, if a scientist has not kept abreast of current research with informal contacts available through his employment, he may be as much as 2 years outdated even if he has a new PhD.

The scientist makes a choice when he takes his first job. If he goes into industry or government, his chances for subsequent academic employment, with its higher prestige, are very small. If he remains within the academic world, however, he can expect little difficulty in shifting to industry or government employment later, should he so desire. Many scientists have moved from academic to partial employment in industrial areas as a result of inventions developed from their academic work.

The highly successful academic scientist generally becomes an entrepreneur with a laboratory of several other scientists, postdoctoral students, graduate students, and so on. He will frequently move into a position that involves more administration than research.

Scientists who want to remain within the scientific community and within the group of researchers active in basic research problems will stay employed either in a university setting or in an exceptional outside laboratory. There they are best able to communicate with other scientists, publish, and work on problems of interest to them and to the scientific community.

Adapted from Nicholas C. Mullins, *Science: Some Sociological Perspectives.* © 1973 by the Bobbs-Merrill Company, Inc.

15. The author's assertion that scientists "age" is most accurately meant to illustrate:

A. the need to constantly recruit younger, more enthusiastic scientists into both academic as well as industrial positions.
B. the importance of being an active member of scientific communities.
C. the importance of being conceptually flexible in one's work.
D. the need for scientists to recognize their own obsolescence.

16. Based on information in the passage, unemployment for scientists is largely attributable to:

A. constant and rapid changes in scientific knowledge.
B. the inability of scientists to coordinate both professional and administrative responsibilities.
C. the inability of scientists to establish and maintain informal contacts through their employment.
D. overreliance on outdated conceptual schemes.

17. The connection between scientific work and prestige is characterized by the author as being based on:

A. the early career decisions of scientists.
B. a professional reliance on other researchers in an entrepreneurial setting.
C. avoiding the difficulties in shifting from an academic to an industrial setting.
D. the centrality of professional publications.

18. Based on the logic of the passage, the author appears to make concerted efforts to:

A. discourage most aspiring scientists from entering the field.
B. encourage potential scientists to make intelligent career choices.
C. encourage most scientists to pursue administrative or instructional positions.
D. all of the above.

19. According to the author, which of the following topics should be the scientist's highest priority?

A. Professional affiliations
B. University employment
C. Professional publications
D. Entrepreneurial skills

20. According to the author, which of the following topics should be the scientist's lowest priority?

A. Administrative duties
B. Industry employment
C. Informal contacts
D. Professional publications

Passage IV (Questions 21–27)

A noted sociologist recently reported the results of a 10-year study on homelessness. The sociologist came to some grim conclusions about the existence of compassion in the United States. I agree with his findings. Despite the fact that he noted the occasional gesture of kindness, he is convinced that the streets of America will forever be populated by people for whom we have little or no concern. And the most frightening aspect is not simply that we refuse to help those now on the streets, but that there are so many very poor waiting to take their places. And those in wait are terrified.

And they should be terrified, for I have met many who inhabit the alleys, doorways, and whatever urban aperture that presents some measure of safety or comfort—as if these two qualities could be counted as realities in their particular world. The streets are frightening, dangerous, and intimidating places. Considering the fact that the average American with a permanent residence now fears venturing out alone, particularly at night, one can hardly imagine the anxieties experienced by our fellow Americans who can boast of no address. I am angered by the stereotypes offered of the homeless, characterizing them as dangerous and overwhelmingly criminal in intent. Few realize that the homeless are far more often the victims of crime than the perpetrators—victims of innumerable robberies, thousands of rapes, and just as many murders. Adding to the atrocity of the situation is the fact that many of these people, if not most, are never reported to the police, and should the authorities become involved, efforts at "solving" the crime or bringing the criminals to justice are halfhearted at best. Our authorities appear to share the same sense of complacency as the average citizen: Who cares? And of course, who is going to demand that police investigations are thorough and efficient? Certainly not the other homeless, who are more often just as frightened by encounters with the police as they are by any other aspect of street life.

Fear for personal safety is far more central to the psychological and physical existence of the homeless than we acknowledge. Of course, many of us regiment our lives to avoid compromising or potentially dangerous situations. And in doing so, we purchase firearms, install security alarms, lock our doors, or simply stay home. The measure of comfort provided by a home, an apartment, or even a hotel room is extraordinary, but it is something we all too often take for granted. Indeed, the importance of our homes, our sanctums, becomes all too evident when we are somehow denied access. Think of your own panic the last time you were unable to find your house key. Trees, park benches, and parking garages certainly present no such problems; however, they do provide for exposure, vulnerability, and easy victimization.

Understanding the experience of homelessness demands that we acknowledge such realities. Homelessness is, in fact, very hard work. I do understand that most of us toil diligently and conscientiously in mainstream forms of employment. But the simple fact is that homelessness as an existence is far more difficult and exceedingly more dangerous than anything that the majority of the gainfully employed will ever know. Dealing with ever-present difficulty and danger requires overwhelming effort and expertise. Unfortunately, few of us pay attention to these facts and, as such, think of the homeless as little more than irresponsible and unworthy. And this is precisely why we will not care. Further, we continue to attribute to these human beings those seemingly (and inevitably?) associated qualities, such as alcoholism, hostility, and mental illness—as if being homeless were essentially a package deal. Well, here I must agree. Unfortunately, the contents of this package more often come from the experience of being homeless than the other way around. Were I to spend months, if not years, on the streets, I too would drink, become antisocial, and suffer psychologically. If I am not mistaken, were such things as alcoholism and even irresponsibility truly the causes of homelessness, things in this country would be far, far worse.

21. The experience of homelessness in the United States tends to be misunderstood by most Americans because they:

A. rarely see the homeless in a positive light.
B. tend to assume that most homeless men and women are criminals.
C. rarely see the homeless as responsible and worthy human beings.
D. fail to recognize the skills the homeless actually possess.

22. The author's discussion of life on the streets of America suggests that:

A. particularly at night, most Americans tend to avoid being on the streets altogether.
B. most Americans do not truly understand the causes of homelessness.
C. being homeless can, in fact, change people.
D. alcoholism, hostility, and mental illness are relatively commonplace.

23. The discussion of crime in the passage best illustrates the author's point that:

A. the police investigate crimes against the domiciled far more efficiently and thoroughly.
B. the homeless are consistently being victimized by the nonhomeless.
C. the homeless are most often honest and hardworking individuals.
D. the relationship between crime and homelessness is completely misunderstood.

24. From the reasoning presented in the passage, which of the following statements would the author be most likely to make?

A. Social services, such as alcohol, drug, and mental health programs, need to be dramatically expanded in the United States.
B. Most Americans overestimate their likelihood of being a victim of crime.
C. Most Americans underestimate their relative advantages.
D. Most Americans could be considered relatively irresponsible.

25. When the author speaks of the inefficiency and halfhearted efforts of the police in investigating crimes involving the homeless, a key link is established between these efforts and:

A. the powerlessness of the homeless.
B. the carelessness of the authorities.
C. the complacency of the homeless.
D. the ineptitude of the homeless.

26. The passage reference to the "many very poor waiting" to take the places of the homeless in the United States implies that:

A. most Americans are very close to being homeless.
B. there exists a very fine line between being homeless and being domiciled.
C. the conditions of poverty in America are extremely precarious.
D. most poor Americans expect to spend at least part of their lives on the streets.

27. When the author appears to agree with the views of the average American, it is:

A. based on an acknowledgment of the pervasiveness of substance abuse on the streets.
B. based on an acknowledgment of the psychological distress engendered by homelessness.
C. purely superficial and actually demonstrates the author's use of sarcasm.
D. meant to make the reader aware of his own irresponsibility.

Passage V (Questions 28–34)

The similarity of one mythology to another may be owed to the growth of similar conditions of society. Its character must vary based on the tribe in which it originates. The ferocious tribe, collecting skulls of slaughtered enemies, must have a very different mythology from that of a peaceful tribe, loitering away hours in idle pastimes.

At a later and more refined period, we sometimes find these primitive legends combined into a regular system under the hands of the poet. The rude outline becomes molded into forms of ideal beauty, which are the objects of adoration in a credulous age and the delight of all succeeding ones. Such were the beautiful inventions of Hesiod and Homer, who say the Father of History "created the theogony of the Greeks"; an assertion not to be taken too literally because it is hardly possible that any man should create a religious system for his nation. They only filled up the shadowy outlines of tradition with the bright touches of their own imaginations, until they had clothed them in beauty that kindled the imaginations of others. The power of the poet, indeed, may be felt in a similar way in a much riper period of society. To say nothing of the "Divina Commedia," who is there that rises from the perusal of "Paradise Lost" without feeling his own conceptions of the angelic hierarchy quickened by those of the inspired artist, and a new and sensible form, as it were, given to images which have before floated dim and undefined before him?

The last mentioned period is succeeded by that of philosophy, which disclaiming alike the legends of the primitive age and the poetical embellishments of the succeeding one, seeks to shelter itself from the charge of impiety. It does this by giving an allegorical interpretation to the popular mythology and, thus, to reconcile the latter with the genuine deductions of science.

The civil policy of the Aztecs was so closely blended with their religion that, without understanding the latter, it is impossible to form correct ideas of their government or their social institutions.

The Mexican religion has emerged from the first of the periods we have been considering. Although little affected by poetical influences, the Mexican religion was controlled by the priests, who had digested as thorough and burdensome a ceremonial as ever existed in any nation. They had, moreover, thrown the veil of allegory over early tradition and invested their deities with attributes, savoring much more of the lighter fictions of Greek mythology, in which the features of humanity, however exaggerated, were never wholly abandoned.

In contemplating the religious system of the Aztecs, one is struck with comparatively refined people, open to gentle influences, whereas the rest breathe a spirit of unmitigated ferocity. It naturally suggests the idea of two distinct sources and authorizes the belief that the Aztecs had inherited from their predecessors a milder faith, on which was afterwards engrafted their own mythology. The latter soon become dominant and gave its dark coloring to the creeds of the conquered nations—which the Mexicans, as the ancient Romans, seem willingly to have incorporated into their own—until the same funeral superstition settled over the farthest borders of Anahuac.

Adapted from E. D. Morgan, *The Key to Unlocking Ancient Societies.* © 1995 by E. D. Morgan

28. The author of the passage would agree with which of the following statements?

I. Religious myth is shaped by environment.
II. Religious myth is shaped by literature.
III. Religious myth is shaped by philosophy.

A. I and III only
B. II and III only
C. I only
D. I and II only

29. The author's attitude toward the claim that Hesiod and Homer created the Greek religion can be best described as:

A. incredulous.
B. bemused.
C. skeptical.
D. affirmative.

30. The word *philosophy* in paragraph three of the passage carries a meaning most similar to the word:

A. rationalism.
B. ethics.
C. literary criticism.
D. atheism.

31. According to the author, the ancient Aztec religion was:

A. highly embellished with poetical tales.
B. similar to the Greek religion in its conception of deity.
C. dichotomous in makeup or outlook.
D. narrow in geographic influence.

32. The passage supports the idea that the Aztec influence on Mexican religious tradition was one of greater:

I. rationality.
II. ferocity.
III. abstraction.

A. I and III only
B. III only
C. II and III only
D. II only

33. The passage implies that the Mexican gods were:

A. man-like.
B. irreconcilable.
C. similar in some respects to Asian deities.
D. similar in some respects to Greek deities.

34. The author justifies the study of ancient religion by:

A. claiming that only in this way can ancient societies be understood.
B. asserting that all knowledge is good for its own sake.
C. expressing anxiety that otherwise there might be deviations from scriptural truth.
D. making the observation that ancient religions and Christianity are often similar.

Passage VI (Questions 35–42)

For years, people have argued that criminals are best understood as products of their environments and that most crime is the result of poverty, poor child rearing, or other numerous seemingly pathological conditions. These explanations have received a great deal of attention from politicians, academics, and social workers alike. Unfortunately, although these attempts to understand are well-grounded in sound social and scientific research, they appear to neglect the importance of something else—the seductive qualities of crime itself. Criminal behavior most certainly results from conditions of extreme poverty as well as poor parenting; however, to assume that crime and one's background are inevitably connected assumes a sentimentality that needs to be challenged. This challenge is rather easy based on some very simple observations. For example, most of the poor do not commit crimes, whereas many wealthy, well-established individuals do. There is little doubt that seemingly "well-adjusted" men and women commonly are indicted for committing heinous acts against others. And in these situations, because their actions cannot be so easily connected to background, we are quick to jump to some explanation of their pathological psychological tendencies long hidden from the eyes of either family members or therapists.

By relying heavily on background to explain crime, we have neglected the foreground of criminal activity itself. What this means is that there is very often something that occurs in immediate situations that, regardless of from where we come and who are our parents, compels us to do things that cannot be explained in such convenient terms. This does not mean that seemingly hidden pathological conditions surface in times of crisis or anxiety, but that specific forms of interaction with other human beings often evoke extraordinary responses. One need only think about a situation in which one appeared to "overreact" to make a point. Think for the moment about "going overboard" and suddenly being confronted with the fact that you could not believe you did something you did.

All too often analysts tend to overlook the fact that human beings, regardless of class, ethnicity, or gender, find themselves in situations that challenge not these status variables but the very moral existence of the person involved. By moral existence, I refer to their status as individuals irrespective of background; their status based on such important moral emotions as dignity, self-esteem, and competence. Take, for example, the driver who is driven to the side of the road by another, or the thief who is confronted by an indignant victim. In both cases, what is most often central is neither a concern for observing the rules of the road nor the pathology of the assailant, but rather the defense of one's self as a competent and valuable human being. To this extent, to speak of crime as being the consequence of background is quite simply a mistake. Thus, the driver who pulls out a gun or the thief who ultimately but unintentionally murders a victim does so not specifically because of who they are, but because of where they are and what they are experiencing at that point in time.

In trying to understand crime, we need to move beyond the sentimental academic attachments of the past and pay greater attention to the immediacy of the situation. This means that criminological research must also involve an exploration of the interactional dynamics in which individuals find themselves, rather than concentrating on such things as alcoholic mothers and failed educational experiences. Once again, background most certainly matters; however, the predictive qualities of these factors need to be complemented by a deeper understanding of what more immediately drives men and women to do what they do. Very often, to speak of irrational behaviors or cold-blooded murder also appears to miss the point completely. In a detailed and more carefully considered analysis, what they have done may indeed be hideous but may also make perfect sense.

35. According to the passage, efforts to explain crime based on such things as poverty and poor child-rearing practices reflect:

A. poorly grounded social scientific explanations of criminal behavior.
B. a limited approach to understanding the causes of crime in America.
C. completely misguided efforts to understand criminality in the United States.
D. all of the above.

36. According to the passage, the challenge to traditional efforts at understanding crime is based largely on which of the following statements?

A. The disillusionment with the state of criminology itself
B. Newly discovered information about the pathology of criminals
C. The need to understand the more contemporary elements of criminality
D. The range of individuals who actually commit crimes

37. Based on information in the passage, the real difference between criminals who come from poorer backgrounds and wealthier offenders is:

A. the nature of the crimes that each individual is likely to commit.
B. first and foremost a function of motive.
C. difficult to distinguish because of our traditional preoccupation with the crimes of the poor.
D. negligible because of the dynamics of crime itself.

38. Based on the fact that the number of violent crimes in the United States is decreasing, the author would most likely argue that:

A. the conditions of poverty in the United States are effectively being remedied.
B. this decrease can only be partially attributed to improving social conditions.
C. Americans appear to have become relatively more law abiding.
D. the treatment of pathological conditions contributing to crime appears successful.

39. Which of the following statements best supports the general argument made in the passage?

A. To an extent, there is no fundamental psychological difference between criminals and noncriminals.
B. The psychological makeup of most criminals is relatively consistent.
C. Reliance on psychological explanations of crime tends to exaggerate the distinction between criminals and non-criminals.
D. Most, if not all, Americans are potential criminals.

40. Which of the following observations provides the strongest challenge to the logic presented in the passage?

A. Of all the murders committed in the United States each year, more than 50% involve African-American men killing other African-American men.
B. The majority of murders committed in the United States each year involve people who know each other intimately.
C. Murders committed by women almost always involve the killing of intimates.
D. Despite the fact that the United States has the highest murder rate in the world, murder is still a relatively rare event.

41. The example of the driver who seemingly "overreacts" is used by the author to argue that:

A. Americans tend to overvalue such things as dignity and self-esteem.
B. situational dynamics may lead usually law-abiding citizens to act in an extreme manner.
C. Americans tend to overreact to challenges to self-esteem and competence.
D. situational dynamics may cause usually law-abiding citizens to overvalue such things as dignity and self-esteem.

42. According to the author, references to such things as "irrational behavior" and "cold-blooded murder" as relatively useless implies that:

A. these terms can be used to explain only a limited proportion of the crimes committed in the United States.
B. these terms fail to address the fact that crime may well be the result of human beings who are generally competent individuals.
C. victims of crime very often play a central role in their own victimization.
D. most crimes can be explained relatively easily.

Passage VII (Questions 43–48)

I hated learning to drive. The entire experience involved not only tremendous peer pressure to get a driver's license, but also the anxiety and agony of dealing with my father's preoccupation with fastidious conduct while on the road. I wanted to drive, but in retrospect, it's clear to me that the demands so often placed on a 16-year-old adolescent now appear completely unwarranted. To be able to drive, to have one's driver's license, is, in a sense, a proclamation of freedom. At the same time, however, it also seems to have been one more submission to the dictates of parental control. Psychologically, a license may well be liberating, but in purely familial terms, it always seemed to provide one more excuse for my parents to dictate the terms of my life. Is this tension simply part of adolescence? If so, I would suggest that parents inform their children of the hazards they are about to encounter off the road as well as on it.

I know that I failed my first two driving tests because of the fears instilled by my examiner, my father, and my friends who expected new and wonderful doors to open upon my success and through my newly found freedom. Yet having finally received my license, it appeared as though my freedom was, in fact, to be highly compromised. Not only was I at the mercy of my parents, who owned the automobiles I might drive, but I was also at the mercy of my friends who successively determined where I would go and what I would do in those vehicles. Where exactly I was located in these decision-making processes still escapes me, and to this day I feel compelled to ask where I am going and what I am to do before I put the key into the ignition.

As a result, I am also compelled, if not completely fascinated, by those men and women who find driving a liberating experience. I wonder how and why these individuals learned to drive. Surely they must have taken it upon themselves to steal the keys of some unwitting car owner and steal into the night on some back country road. How else could they possibly have been spared the agony of the screams and admonitions of well-meaning and experienced overseers? To this extent, I am an adamant advocate of "borrowing" your parents' car while they visit grandmother and seeing what transpires. At the very least, any unanticipated collisions are undoubtedly attributable to inexperience rather than to the fear of the wrath of one's instructor. As far as I am concerned, far fewer "instructional" accidents would ever plague our highways if would-be drivers were driven to learn (excuse the pun) by more purely personal initiative and were taught by complete strangers.

To this end I would ask that all potential drivers exercise the greatest caution in their decisions to become masters of the road. Most importantly, I would suggest that they learn to drive for personal reasons alone and that they seek instruction from a genuinely disinterested party. Do not learn to drive from someone upon whom you must rely to continue your pursuits, and do not learn to drive to satisfy the interests of another. To do so will inevitably lead to a driving career fraught with anxiety and, without a doubt, more tickets for moving violations than you would ever expect or desire. To drive at the age of 16 years because one feels compelled to do so is usually a mistake. Learn to drive because you want to, not because of the demands of being a teenager. People often point amusingly at 30-year-old individuals who take the bus or rely on taxis to get around. Perhaps we should applaud these individuals who have had the conviction to avoid driving altogether.

43. The passage suggests that, for most teenagers, learning to drive is:

A. inevitably connected to learning to become independent.
B. something to be feared and avoided altogether.
C. little more than a rite of passage.
D. best described as a struggle for independence.

44. According to the passage, the liberating effects of driving for teenagers are usually most highly compromised by which of the following demands?

A. The demands placed on the individual to demonstrate competence as a driver
B. The demands placed on the individual to deal with the trials of instruction
C. The demands placed on the individual that restrict self-control over his or her driving
D. The demands placed on the individual to exercise good judgment as a driver

45. Based on information in the passage, the best driver would be the individual who:

A. consistently challenges those who dictate the terms of his or her driving.
B. relies more heavily on public transportation than anything else.
C. drives as infrequently as possible.
D. is essentially self-taught.

46. The characterization of peer pressure in the passage suggests primarily that most teenagers are:

A. highly influenced by the need to be accepted by friends.
B. unfairly forced to contend with the demands of peers.
C. constantly forced to balance the demands of peers with those of parents.
D. basically unthinking and obedient to the demands of others.

47. In the passage, the biggest source of confusion for the author appears to be the:

A. genuine reasons behind having learned to drive.
B. general preoccupation in this country with the need to drive.
C. purposes of driving.
D. traditional role of the driver in the act of driving.

48. In consideration of the passage, the fact that there are more cars in the United States than any other nation in the world suggests that:

A. the author appears to misunderstand the importance of driving.
B. the pressures to drive in this country are indeed overwhelming.
C. Americans tend to overestimate the need to drive.
D. the author's anxieties about driving appear purely personal.

Passage VIII (Questions 49–56)

The suffering caused by AIDS is enormous. Sufferers deserve compassion, and their disease deserves scientific inquiry. But AIDS has got far more. AIDS has become the most privileged disease in America. Why? Mainly because its victims are young and, in many cases, creative and famous. Their deaths are therefore particularly poignant and public. Another reason is because some of the groups that AIDS disproportionately affects are highly organized. This combination of conspicuousness and constituency has allowed AIDS activists to get more research funding, more treatment money, and looser drug-testing restrictions than any comparable disease.

There is nothing wrong with that. The system for allocating research and treatment money in American medicine is archaic, chaotic, and almost random anyway. Under the "Disease-of-the-Month-Club" syndrome, any disease that has in some way affected a Congressman or some relation gets special treatment. There is rough justice in this method of allocation because after a while Congressmen and their kin get to experience most of the medical tragedies that life has to offer. At the end of the day, therefore, funds tend to get allocated in a fairly proportionate way.

AIDS is now riding a crest of public support, won in the rough and tumble of politics. This is all perfectly legitimate and is a tribute to the passion and commitment of AIDS activists. But that passion turns to a mere stridency when they take to the streets to protest that a phobic society has been ungenerous and stinting in its response to the tragedy of AIDS. In fact, American society is giving overwhelming and indeed disproportionate attention and resources to the fight.

At first, the afflicted communities were disoriented and defensive in reaction to AIDS. In the quite understandable attempt to get public support, they fixed on a strategy of claiming that AIDS was everyone's problem. Because we were all potential sufferers—"Anyone can get AIDS," went the slogan—society as an act of self-protection should go all out for cure and care.

This campaign was initially successful. But then it ran into an obstacle. It was somewhat misleading that AIDS was everyone's problem. The AIDS activists, therefore, now appeal less to solidarity than to guilt: every person who dies is more blood on the hands of a society unwilling to give every dollar demanded for a cure.

But society has blood on its hands every time it refuses to give every dollar demanded by the cancer, heart disease, and diabetes lobbies. So now a different tack: the claim that the AIDS epidemic is, of course, not an act of government but an act of nature, and government has not done enough to help its helpless victims.

In fact, AIDS is far less an act of nature than is, say, cancer or diabetes. Apart from a small number of relentlessly exploited Ryan White-like exceptions, the overwhelming majority of sufferers get AIDS through voluntary action. You do not get AIDS the way you used to get tuberculosis (TB), by having someone in the subway cough in a crowded place. You do not get it the way you get, say, brain cancer, which is through some act of nature that we do not understand at all.

From Charles Krauthammer, "America's Response to AIDS Is Adequate" in ***Current Controversies: The Aids Crisis.***

49. The general tone of the passage appears to be:

A. frustration and indignation at the efforts of AIDS activists.

B. a carefully qualified acceptance of the efforts of AIDS activists.

C. in clear opposition to the efforts of AIDS activists.

D. generally in sympathy with the efforts of AIDS activists.

50. According to the author, the current state of AIDS funding is most accurately the result of:

A. archaic and chaotic efforts to allocate research dollars.
B. a traditionally high level of public support.
C. specific and influential members of Congress.
D. high-profile casualties of the disease.

51. On the basis of the author's observations about the political strategies of AIDS activists, it is reasonable to conclude that the author believes the future of AIDS funding is likely to:

A. remain high because of the epidemic nature of the disease.
B. decline because of the epidemiological characteristics of the disease.
C. remain high because of public misunderstandings about the disease.
D. decline because of competition from other political lobbyists.

52. The discussion of phobia in the passage is used to illustrate which of the following topics?

A. The pervasiveness of hostile attitudes toward gay men and women in America
B. The apprehension of most Americans to support funding for AIDS
C. The loud and obtrusive quality of AIDS activism
D. The passionate nature of AIDS activism

53. According to the passage, the suggestion that AIDS is not everyone's problem likely means that:

A. diseases contracted through intentional actions deserve far less attention than those contracted unintentionally.
B. the connection of AIDS to specific forms of behavior and drug use needs to be an important consideration in the allocation of research and treatment money.
C. campaigns for research and treatment dollars may be inappropriately influenced by misinformation of public risk.
D. A, B, and C

54. The author could strongly support a research funding process based on the allocation of research and treatment dollars:

A. irrespective of the characteristics of affected populations.
B. proportionate to the numbers of persons affected.
C. irrespective of the notoriety of persons affected.
D. irrespective of the age of affected populations.

55. The mention of "rough justice" in the passage is most accurately meant to describe the:

A. fact that members of Congress are by no means exempt from the tragedies we must all face.
B. indignation of the author at the political nature of research and treatment funding.
C. indignation of the author at the arbitrary nature of research and treatment funding.
D. ultimate but indirect equitableness in the allocation of research and treatment dollars.

56. Which of the following statements best describes the author's overall objective in this passage?

A. Current funding for AIDS treatment and research is simply too great and needs to be reevaluated.
B. Political strategies are central to the success of demands for research money.
C. AIDS sufferers need to assume more of the financial burden for research and treatment.
D. There are other high-profile diseases being neglected in the allocation of research and treatment dollars for AIDS.

Passage IX (Questions 57–65)

Standard pharmacological definitions of the term *drug* nearly always run something like this: "any substance (other than food) that, by its chemical or physical nature, alters structure or function in the living organism." This sounds quite reasonable at first, but some reflection renders it meaningless and without utility. By this definition, water would be a drug; so would oxygen. Almost any chemical substance has an effect on living tissue; so do a wide range of activities. In fact, almost nothing whatsoever has no effect at all on the human organism.

Granted that the standard pharmacological definition is far too broad to be useful, is it possible to arrive at a meaningful objective definition of drugs? Is there any characteristic that groups together all, or nearly all, substances that would more or less universally be regarded as drugs, while unambiguously excluding those that almost no one would want to call drugs? The answer is no. Some drugs are physically "addicting" (i.e., produce a cellular dependence in the organism), whereas others are not. Some drugs are toxic and lethal; others are not capable of killing humans in the doses typically taken even by the heaviest users. Some drugs are psychoactive; others have little effect on the way we think and feel, on the processes of the human mind and psyche. In fact, running down any roster of possible drug effects, it becomes clear that there is no formal property that is simultaneously (1) shared by more or less all drug substances and also (2) alien to nondrug substances.

And yet, all this time, I have been using the term *drug*. If an objective definition is impossible, does this mean that the word is useless? No; what it means is that instead of searching inside drugs for their intrinsic properties and biochemical reactions (which drugs supposedly touch off), something that all drugs "do," it is necessary to search outside the substances themselves, to see how they are defined, used, and conceptualized. A drug is anything that is defined as a drug.

Definitions will differ, mainly according to the purpose for making the decision in the first place. A policeman or someone reading the morning newspaper will think of drugs primarily in legal terms: substances whose possession is against the law. Within this definition, marijuana, cocaine, heroin, and LSD would be drugs. But a physician might think of drugs primarily in therapeutic terms: substances used in conjunction with healing. Then penicillin, antibiotics, digitalis, and steroids would be drugs. If we are concerned with the psychoactive side of chemicals and think of drugs as substances that have an impact on the functioning of the human mind, then we would think of alcohol, marijuana, LSD, and mescaline as drugs, but penicillin would not be so regarded. There are, of course, countless other ways of defining and looking at chemical substances as "drugs." What we call a drug is arbitrary and depends on our purposes for making the categorization in the first place. In short, the category "drug" is humanly fabricated. What is or is not a drug is decided not by nature, but by us, by humans—by definition.

From Erich Goode, *The Drug Phenomenon: Social Aspects of Drug Taking.* © 1973 by The Bobbs-Merrill Company, Inc.

57. According to the passage, standard pharmacological definitions of drugs tend to be useless because such definitions:

A. claim to be objective in nature.
B. fail to distinguish between the effects of different types of drugs.
C. are almost always overly inclusive.
D. fail to acknowledge both medical and legal definitions.

58. The author of the text appears to suggest that conventional wisdom about drugs is based on:

A. little or no scientific evidence.
B. faulty scientific knowledge.
C. illogical scientific reasoning.
D. misguided scientific expertise.

59. The author's statement that "there is no formal property that is simultaneously shared by more or less all drug substances and also alien to nondrug substances" assumes that the scientific category of "drugs" is:

A. essentially meaningless.
B. essentially nonexistent.
C. effectively nonexclusive.
D. effectively nonscientific.

60. Which of the following claims made in the passage is the LEAST supported?

A. The scientific categorization of drugs fails to reflect any objective reality.
B. The definition of drugs is inevitably linked to interests.
C. There are countless ways of defining drugs.
D. Legal definitions are just as relevant as scientific definitions.

61. Based on the information in the passage, which of the following opinions could be most reasonably ascribed to the author?

A. Legal sanctions against those who use illicit drugs need to be eliminated.
B. The distinction between licit and illicit drugs is meaningless.
C. Legal sanctions against those who use illicit drugs need to be relaxed.
D. The distinction between licit and illicit drugs is largely political.

62. Recent proposals in the United States calling for the legalization of marijuana for medical purposes would be considered by the author to be justified because:

A. of the ambiguity of scientific research on drugs.
B. the categorization of marijuana as illicit is completely unfounded.
C. marijuana cannot reasonably be classified as a drug.
D. of the potential benefits of marijuana for the chronically ill.

63. Which of the following statements most strongly supports the general theme of the passage?

A. Morphine and heroin are essentially the same chemical substance and differ basically in legal terms alone.
B. Cigarette smoking is just as harmful, if not more so, than the use of many illicit drugs in the United States.
C. There exists no fundamentally important difference between crack cocaine and powdered cocaine.
D. The use of steroids among professional athletes is commonplace.

64. According to the logic of the passage, the term *drug abuse* would probably refer to:

A. the development of a drug addiction.
B. the heavy use of psychoactive drugs.
C. the value judgments of interested parties.
D. the subjective definition of a drug user.

65. The author's disregard for the importance of understanding the intrinsic properties of drugs is based on which of the following assumptions?

A. It is essentially impossible to understand the intrinsic qualities of most drugs.
B. Knowing the intrinsic qualities of drugs tells us little about their effects.
C. The intrinsic properties of drugs are highly variable.
D. All of the above.

Solutions to Verbal Reasoning Practice Test 2

PASSAGE I

1. **D** According to information in the passage, the central theme is that of (largely) political opinions that make constant reference to concerns over maintaining the identity of the United States as an English-speaking nation. Indeed, these concerns are extended to beliefs about English becoming the "next world language." Thus, references to schooling, territorial settlements, and the adjustment of immigrants lend themselves best to choice D. Choice A is touched on by the author in the closing lines of the passage; however, this hardly constitutes the central theme of the passage. In fact, when the author does make reference to potential problems here, it is still not stated with as much conviction as choice A implies. Choice B might seem reasonable; however, the passage does not trace actual efforts to establish English as the official language of the country and, therefore, can also be eliminated. Choice C can also be eliminated for the reason that, to this day, English is not the official language of the United States.
2. **C** Based on the information in the passage and the tone of the author, no definite convictions are put forth regarding the controversy over the use of English or whether or not its establishment as official is necessarily good or bad. Therefore, it seems clear that the author is relatively indifferent to efforts to privilege the use of English in the United States. Based on the information above, choices A, B, and D are all easily eliminated. Indeed, the author expresses some skepticism about forcing others to learn a language; however, this is not necessarily expressed as fear or a definite challenge to such efforts.
3. **D** Following information from question one, the passage points to historical efforts to privilege English rather than make it official. Also, from the information provided, these efforts have been relatively indirect in terms of actual strategies. The reader should consider the limited information about the settlement of English speakers in newly acquired territories and even challenges to territorial acquisition based on language concerns, both of which are more indirect efforts at language protection. While the passage does note some obvious examples of racism, there is no evidence that actual efforts have been made to deny language rights. In fact, the school decision cited upheld foreign language instruction in schools. Therefore, choice A can be eliminated. Choice B draws attention to xenophobia; however, there is no evidence here of actual legislation along these lines. Choice C may seem reasonable, yet no territorial acquisitions appear to have actually been prevented based on concerns over language.
4. **D** The general conclusion of the passage appears to be that the assimilation and adjustment of immigrants is the greatest concern to the

United States. Although other "fears" and assumptions are noted, they are singular examples of a more general attitude. Choice A looks reasonable; however, there is little evidence suggesting that communication with English speakers is the most important concern here. In fact, interaction with non-English speakers is not even directly addressed in the passage, particularly in terms of it being potentially threatening. Choice B is easily eliminated in that the only reference to language instruction in schools is not enhanced by any concerted challenge to such rights. Choice C is actually cited as a singular example and is, in fact, used by the author to state a rather extreme position.

5. **B** Based on information in the final lines of the passage, the author simply notes his own skepticism regarding efforts to force the learning of a second language. To this extent, his observations suggest the difficulties of such endeavors based on generally disappointing experiences in schools and the furor often connected to efforts at bilingual education. Choice A may well be true; however, it is certainly not substantiated by information in the passage. In fact, it may well overstate the opposition to other languages. Choice C can be eliminated because the author generally avoids being judgmental about efforts to privilege English. In fact, this choice tends to overstate the milder skepticism that the author demonstrates in the passage. Choice D is flawed for similar reasons and makes a sweeping generalization that is, once again, not substantiated in the passage.

6. **A** Based largely on information provided in the second paragraph of the passage, the most reasonable choice is A. The passage notes that most Americans assume that the rest of the world either does or should speak English. At the same time, the paragraph does not specifically point to partial efforts at speaking English or efforts to learn to do so. Extending the information above, the passage notes that "Americans often assume that all the world speaks English, or that it should." No other qualifications are offered here, and, although choices B and C appear to be reasonable extensions of these observations, no such evidence is offered in the passage. Therefore, choice A is still the best answer. Choice D represents an extreme attitude toward other languages but is evidenced by a singular historical statement and cannot be extended to the average American.

7. **C** Because the tone of the passage is generally neutral, it seems safest to assume that the author wishes to note his skepticism about potential efforts to privilege English, but that he is relatively uncertain about the future of such efforts. Therefore, it seems reasonable to state that the future of language legislation is best described as ambiguous. Choice A is simply not substantiated by information in the passage. Although the author makes a general observation about what "may . . . always be the basic human condition," this is not necessarily easily generalized to the American experience. Choice B may well be true but, once again, nothing in the passage points to this inevitability.

The same can be said of choice D. The elimination of these last two choices is based largely on the lack of sufficient information.

PASSAGE II

8. **A** The contemporary character of Halloween appears to be the most obvious concern considering the author's reference to "the recklessness commonly associated with it" and "the fears for the safety of children." The emphasis of the passage is clearly on the current worries that Americans appear to harbor. Choice A notes the historical roots of Halloween, but the author notes that "we now emphasize the fantastical side" of the holiday rather than the origins of Halloween. Choice C addresses the psychological disadvantages; however, the psychological advantages are precisely what the author chooses to emphasize in the defense of celebrating Halloween. Choice D is relatively meaningless here, and the relevance of anthropology is apparent only in that the explanation of an anthropologist is chosen to support the author's observations.

9. **C** The essence of the passage is that Americans somehow are allowed, through the celebration of Halloween, to confront their fears. Note the author's reference to the fact that Halloween allows us to "control unruly characters or attitudes that may frighten or intrigue," and, thus, we gain from this manipulation rather than lose. Therefore, the relationship between what we fear and the celebration of the holiday essentially is advantageous. Choice A assumes that Americans misunderstand the holiday, but this is countered by the fact that the author notes "we relish and understand the value" of what we do on Halloween. Choice B is unacceptable on these same terms. Choice D is based solely on the reference to the efforts of school boards cited as examples of attempts to ban the holiday and have little relevance for the general population.

10. **D** The question asks for the most accurate observation, and, as such, the best choice is the more general observation that social boundaries are fluid and quite simply changeable. It is important to note here that the author makes no real value judgments about the characteristics of social boundaries but notes simply that they are fluid and can indeed change. Based on the fact that the author does not attempt to evaluate social boundaries, then choices A, B, and C are inappropriate. Choice A refers to the weakness of boundaries, choice B notes their rigidity, and choice C speaks to dangerously vague and ambiguous categories. No such judgments are implied by the author in the passage.

11. **C** The point here is that it is the active and conscious efforts of people facilitated by the celebration of Halloween that help to redefine what is acceptable and unacceptable in American society. As a result, fantasy and role reversal provide precisely these benefits in acknowledging and maintaining society's "normal" life. Choice A is inappropriate

because the author never actually addresses threatening forces as active. Rather, the emphasis in the passage is on the reaffirmation of existing boundaries by allowing us to see what might make society come apart; thus, the assumption that these forces constantly and actively threaten is incorrect. Choice B can be eliminated because no references are made to the avoidance of future problems or lawlessness. Halloween may prevent society from coming apart at the seams; however, it does not necessarily prevent crime as it exists in this country. Choice D is not really relevant, despite the fact that similar points are made about the functions of similar holidays in other countries.

12. **A** The final paragraphs of the passage appear to applaud the creativity of Americans in their abilities to use singular days or celebrations such as Halloween in their reaffirmation of the "normal." Note again the "conscious" efforts of individuals and their contributions of "particular visions" to the creation of a "topsy-turvy world." Choice B implies little more than some noncreative psychological underpinning to the holiday and, thus, neglects the control the author implies that people demonstrate during Halloween. Choice C suggests a similar misunderstanding in terms of participation and notes simply some underlying pathology. Choice D is valid but also appears to misstate the related utility of the holiday.

13. **A** As stated in the opening lines of the passage, most Americans appear to be concerned about the recklessness of the holiday and the safety of their children during Halloween. Thus, the only reasonable choice seems to be addressing lawlessness in general. Choice B notes a growing conservatism in the United States, but it would be a mistake to assume that concerns over crime in general are necessarily connected to conservatism or any other political context. Choice C notes concerns over maintaining order in schools, yet this argument is connected to a singular reference or example used by the author to conceptualize the dissatisfaction of one group of individuals with the holiday. As such, its generality is questionable. Choice D is inappropriate because the religious dimensions addressed in the passage have more to do with keeping religion out of schools rather than making efforts to defend it.

14. **C** The author implies in the passage that the problems associated with Halloween are definitely outweighed by its advantages. At the same time, it is important to note that few details are offered here, other than the elaborated benefits themselves. However, the essence of the argument is that the consequences of Halloween are genuinely less threatening. Choices A and B are unsubstantiated; however, neither is noted explicitly by the author here and thus both can be eliminated. Choice D is logically inappropriate.

PASSAGE III

15. **C** The author's reference to "aging" is clearly meant to refer here to becoming "old" in terms of professional expertise. Thus, rather than encouraging the recruitment of younger, more enthusiastic scientists, the point is that scientists need to remain flexible and receptive to developments in their particular fields. Older scientists can clearly remain current if, as the author suggests, they "accept changes in the way in which a conceptual scheme is being modified." Choice A misunderstands the metaphorical point of the reference and is easily eliminated. Choice B appears reasonable; however, the author's point is that being an active member of the scientific community must involve some very specific directives and that being generally active is no guarantee of success. Choice D is inappropriate because, based on the author's observations, obsolescence should be actively avoided rather than simply accepted.

16. **D** Based on information in the passage, the author attributes the unemployment of scientists most specifically, once again, to their inability to "understand and accept changes in one's conceptual field." As such, flexibility is consistently cited as the major component in the success of scientific careers. Choice A is inappropriate here because the author cites the individual scientist's ability to contend with rapid changes in scientific knowledge and, thus, more apparently condemns those who fail to remain current. Choice B can be eliminated because the coordination of professional and administrative duties is only cited as relevant for scientists who have already achieved success and is, in fact, not considered to be a significant obstacle to a successful scientific career. Choice C is inappropriate because the relevance of informal contacts is, in fact, cited as only an avenue for professional success rather than a central basis.

17. **A** In terms of the connection between scientific work and prestige, the author is clear in noting that early career decisions are central. Here the reader should note constant references to primary choices in employment, as well as the possibilities afforded by certain forms of employment for subsequent opportunities. Thus, early career decisions are, according to the author, crucial to the level of prestige any scientist can ever expect. Rather than suggesting that scientists necessarily rely on fellow professionals, the author seems to imply that only highly successful scientists are afforded this luxury. Thus, choice B can be eliminated. Similarly, choice C implies the move from an already relatively lucrative position in academia to industry; one that is apparently the most intelligent and is relatively easy. Choice D may seem reasonable, but considering the information in the passage, it is only cited as the traditional measure of productivity.

18. **B** Considering the tone of the passage, the author appears to be most likely an advocate of intelligent career choices over anything else. Note the author's consistent references to the choice of employment

setting in terms of future advancement. Choice A might seem reasonable because of the relatively discouraging tone of the passage itself. However, it seems more reasonable to assume that the author is trying to encourage potential scientists to follow the most lucrative path of employment. Choice C clearly seems inappropriate considering the fact that administrative positions are rarely an indication of a successful scientific career. Note the author's observations that "they may be good teachers, advisers, citizens, and employees, but they are not [necessarily] productive scientists." Choice D is logically eliminated.

19. **B** As the passage notes, the most lucrative approach to a successful scientific career is that which allows for the greatest opportunities. As such, the tone of the passage suggests that academic employment provides for the greatest mobility, should the scientist wish to move into industry or government employment later in his or her career. In fact, the author cites the example of this ease of movement explicitly. Choice A is, in fact, cited as a secondary aspect of success based on initial decisions made by the scientist. Choice C is, once again, cited as a traditional measure of productivity, but one that is still clearly connected to initial career decisions. Choice D, as well, is seemingly more connected to the actual status of the scientist in the first place.

20. **C** Based on information discussed in the previous question, the relevance of informal contacts would appear to be the most obvious choice here to the extent that it is the least connected to either initial career decisions or other traditional measures of professional productivity. Choice A is connected to both successful as well as less successful careers and, as such, is a poor choice here. Choice B, or industry employment, is clearly regarded by the author as less preferential to academic employment and can also be eliminated. Choice D is cited as traditionally important; however, it is still seemingly importantly connected to other significant career decisions.

PASSAGE IV

21. **D** The passage notes that most Americans misunderstand the homeless because of their failure to acknowledge the "effort and expertise" the homeless possess in contending with the anxieties and dangers of living on the streets. Importantly, the author connects misunderstanding to "missing information" rather than to stereotypes of the homeless themselves. As such, only choice D is appropriate because it notes what Americans do not know. Choices A, B, and C each make reference to a reasonably valid observation about homelessness; however, they are not the bases for misunderstanding, but rather the expressions of it. Negativity, criminality, and irresponsibility are all better understood here as the consequences of misunderstanding rather than sources.

22. **C** A central theme running throughout the passage is that homelessness is genuinely hard work and very demanding, both psychologically as well as physically. The author argues that connected to these hardships are secondary problems, such as hostility and alcoholism. However, these secondary problems are noted as "consequences" rather than "causes" of homelessness, implying that street life does indeed change people. Choice A is valid; however, it is noted only as a point of comparison with the fears of the homeless and is relatively secondary in importance. In fact, one might argue that it is a misstatement of the author's argument in that it overstates the fear of the average American. Choice B may be valid; however, at no point in the passage does the author ever note "causation" itself. In fact, even in the final lines of the passage, the vague reference to cause is made only in passing and without any elaboration. Choice D is inappropriate because although alcoholism and mental illness are mentioned and even validated as realities on the street, no mention is made of prevalence.

23. **D** The discussion of crime in the passage is used primarily to dispel myths about the relationship between homelessness and crime. To this end, the author notes his anger at "stereotypes . . . characterizing them as dangerous and overwhelmingly criminal in intent", thereby furthering the misunderstanding by the average American. Choice A may seem to be implied by contrast; however, no real reference is made here to the efficiency or thoroughness of the police at all. Thus, choice A appears overly speculative. Choice B is inappropriate because although the author notes that the homeless are more likely to be victims of crime rather than perpetrators, no mention is made of who exactly perpetrators are. Choice C is a noble observation; however, simply because the homeless are referred to as often being victims of crime, there is no basis here allowing the reader to assume that they are necessarily honest and hard working.

24. **C** Considering the contents of the passage, it seems most reasonable that the author would be most likely to argue that most Americans underestimate their relative advantages. Note the author's references to the facts that they take their homes for granted and that most of the employed will never know an existence as dangerous as homelessness. Central to the passage is precisely the vulnerability of the homeless and the sanctums to which most Americans can withdraw. Choice A may be a valid observation, but it is never actually addressed by the author despite references to alcoholism and mental illness on the streets. Indeed, there is no real reference to services at all. Choice B may be inferred considering observations about fears of "venturing out"; however, there is no basis here for assuming that these fears are unfounded. Therefore, choice B is inappropriate. Although the author does appear angry with the attitudes of average Americans, choice D is simply not addressed anywhere in the passage.

25. **A** In the discussion of police handling of crimes against the homeless, the author notes importantly that no one is likely to "demand that

the investigations are thorough and efficient," particularly because the homeless fear encounters with the police. Thus, although the sources of the fear are unclear in the passage, the discussion points to the lack of power the homeless have more than anything else. Fear implies some form of power relationship where the homeless are clearly subordinate. Although the authorities may be inefficient in their work, there is no reference made to "carelessness" itself. In fact, the author attributes the nature of investigations more to the complacency of the police rather than to poor work. Carelessness implies arbitrary and unthinking methods, yet the author suggests the police are completely aware of the circumstances, and they simply choose to limit their efforts. Thus, choice B is inappropriate. Choice C can be eliminated because the lack of participation by other homeless is attributed by the author to fear rather than lack of awareness or interest. Choice D should be eliminated here based on the author's argument that most of the homeless are, in fact, made adept by the fact that they must live on the streets.

26. **C** Although several of these choices might seem reasonable, only choice C is appropriate because few details are offered by the author about how and why exactly the very poor actually become homeless. The reference to how precarious or uncertain poverty is the only appropriate choice. Choice A is inappropriate because it addresses all Americans rather than simply the poor. In fact, the author argues that most Americans are relatively advantaged. Choice B can be eliminated for similar reasons in that the centrality of poverty itself is not addressed. Choice D might seem reasonable; however, it also appears to overgeneralize in the absence of detail provided by the author.

27. **B** Where the author does appear to be in agreement with the average American, it is based on a common ground arrived at from two different directions. The author agrees that alcoholism, hostility, and mental illness are realities on the streets. At the same time, he challenges the extent to which we assume that these are causal factors in homelessness. The author reverses the logic here and notes that these characteristics "come from the experience of being homeless," and, thus, the problems are "engendered by homelessness," not necessarily the causes. Choice A can be eliminated here because the author provides no information on the prevalence of these characteristics. Choice C is inappropriate because the agreement is not itself superficial, it is just carefully qualified. And although one might expect a sarcastic tone here, it is not genuinely evident. The author's tone is more accurately described as critical. Choice D is also inappropriate because references to responsibility are made by the author only to challenge assumptions about the irresponsibility of the homeless.

PASSAGE V

28. **D** This is a difficult passage. Be sure to make a mental map of the passage flow. It is also helpful to make a few cursory notes in the margin next to each paragraph, summarizing key ideas. In this passage, the first paragraph clearly states the author's belief that environment (easy or harsh) influences religious myth. Paragraph two discusses how religious myth is shaped by gifted authors, such as Hesiod and Homer. The passage contains no information supporting statement III. Because statements I and II are supported, the only possible choice is D.

29. **C** The second paragraph supports that choice D is not correct. The burden falls on knowing vocabulary and picking the word out of three near synonyms that best describes the author's tone. Although the author is good humored, it is not fair to describe him as bemused. Nor can one say that an author who is in control of his material as firmly as this one is incredulous. The best choice is that the author is skeptical in paragraph two.

30. **A** Nothing in paragraph three supports choice B or D. The passage is not about ethics, and there is no hint that the author has an atheistic stance. Choice C seems initially plausible because the topic is broadly legends and allegorical interpretation, but choice A is closer to the main intentions or argument of the author. Keep in mind that science, an empirical, rational activity, was once called "natural philosophy."

31. **C** Paragraph five shows that choices A and B are incorrect. The sixth paragraph shows that the Aztec religion was used as a colonizing device, so choice D is incorrect. Paragraph six mainly discusses the incongruous double nature of Aztec religious thought. Choice C is the correct choice.

32. **D** Paragraph six, which compares Aztec religion to other religious thought in Mexico, says nothing to support statement I or III. It does, however, strongly support statement II.

33. **C** Paragraph five specifically compares Mexican gods to "grotesque conceptions of the eastern nations of the Old World," which is to say Asian gods. Choice D is specifically denied in this same sentence. The passage presents no evidence for choices A and B. The passage does say that Aztec religion is somewhat incongruous, but it does not say that the concept of deity is incongruous.

34. **A** The passage presents no evidence in support of choice B, C, or D. The opening sentence of the fourth paragraph makes the claim that only by knowing something of Aztec religion can we hope to understand their way of life, their culture.

PASSAGE VI

35. **B** The central message of the passage is precisely that analysts tend to "neglect . . . the seductive qualities of crime itself." As a result, the author wishes to introduce a complementary approach rather than substitute completely an emphasis on the foreground of crime. Thus, existing explanations are considered by the author to be "limited" in their explanatory power, and choice B is the most appropriate answer. Choice A is, in fact, contrary to what the author argues. Such explanations are well grounded in research but provide, once again, only a partial understanding of the "causes" of crime. Choice C suffers the same problem in that it dismisses existing efforts altogether. Choice D is logically inappropriate.

36. **D** The most fundamental challenge offered by the author to existing explanations is precisely that both "wealthy," "well-adjusted" men and women commit crimes and the fact that this runs contrary to general beliefs about the importance of background. Thus, it is the author's inclusion of traditionally unanticipated individuals into the ranks of criminals that provides the most basic challenge here. Although the author feels the need to supplement existing knowledge, it would be unreasonable to assume that he is completely disillusioned with the field. Therefore, choice A appears to be overstated. Choice B is, in fact, contrary to the general argument in that the author wishes to direct attention away from social and psychological pathology altogether. Choice C is inappropriate because the author does not discuss changes in criminality; rather he discusses elements that have been overlooked.

37. **D** Because the passage makes the central point that the importance of background has been emphasized, the author's argument points toward the importance of the foreground. In doing so, the author notes that the dynamics of certain situations can lead just about anyone to do extreme things. To this extent, the difference between poor and wealthy individuals is considered "negligible because of the dynamics of crime itself." To the extent that the nature of the crimes committed by different individuals is not addressed in the text, Choice A can be eliminated. Choice C is inappropriate because motive is, in fact, generally the same for either type of individual. Choice C can be eliminated because the author implies that no such distinction can really be made. Therefore, traditional preoccupation with background has distracted analysts, but not necessarily in the terms the author wishes to emphasize.

38. **B** The recent decrease in violent crimes would logically be attributed by the author to fewer individuals finding themselves in "morally compromising" circumstances. Therefore, the only reasonable answer would be B to the extent that it at least addresses the importance of information beyond existing knowledge about background or psychological pathologies. Choice A can be eliminated because it relies

completely on a preoccupation with background. Choice C may be true but has no basis in that it assumes that crime is most effectively within the control of the individual. Choice D is inappropriate, considering the author's denial of pathology as central to our ability to explain crime in general.

39. **A** Again, following the logic that circumstances can "evoke very extraordinary responses," the author appears to argue that there exists no fundamental difference between criminals and non-criminals. Consider the author's suggestion that the reader remember a situation in which he or she seemingly overreacted and was shocked at what transpired. This is clearly an effort to connect the law-abiding citizen with the actual criminal. Choice B is inappropriate because it addresses consistency in terms of the psychological makeup of criminals without addressing non-criminals. To this extent, the observation actually attributes some form of psychopathology to the criminal—an argument that the author wishes to avoid altogether. Choice C can be eliminated because it makes a point inconsistent with the logic of the passage if the psychology of the immediate situation is taken into account. In fact, looking at the psychological dynamics of interaction more often illustrates, according to the author, that there is no real distinction. Following the logic of the passage, choice D may be true; however, the passage does not really address the issue of potential as explicitly as the existence of traditional distinctions between criminals and non-criminals.

40. **A** The challenge of the passage to existing explanations is based largely on denying the centrality of such background variables as "class, ethnicity, or gender" and, thus, would be best challenged by criminological findings that stress the importance of such status variables. Therefore, choice A is the most appropriate answer because it notes the relevance of both gender and race and even indirectly notes the relevance of class in the commission of murder in the United States. Choice B, rather than emphasizing the importance of background variables, simply addresses the fact that most murders involve persons who know one another intimately. To this extent, this observation most likely supports the author's arguments considering the likelihood of interaction between the participants. Choice C can be eliminated for similar reasons because, although it addresses gender, it points more to the importance of intimacy. Choice D is true but is largely irrelevant in this context in that the author is not concerned with crime rates.

41. **B** The example of the driver who "overreacts" is used effectively to indicate the vulnerability of usually law-abiding citizens to crime when competence and self-esteem are effectively challenged. Choice B is essentially the only choice that addresses dynamics alone without passing some form of value judgment on those dynamics. To this extent, it is more consistent with the "objectivity" of the passage itself. Rather than suggesting that Americans necessarily overvalue such

things, the author wishes to suggest simply that they are important features in our decisions to act. Thus, choice A is inappropriate because of its evaluative nature. Choice C suffers from the same evaluative quality that indirectly suggests that valuing such things is somehow negative in this context. Choice D provides an inappropriate combination of the aspects of both choices A and C.

42. **C** The author's disdain for such terms as "irrational" and "cold-blooded" are most likely based on the terms' disregard for any sense of logic or rationality in crimes that appear senseless. The best choice is C, which makes the point that victims play central roles in providing challenges to the moral existence of offenders. Therefore, what might look senseless or irrational may well be explainable if approached carefully and considerately. Choice A can be eliminated because the author essentially is arguing the uselessness of the terms themselves. Therefore, it would be a mistake to argue that the authors sees even a limited application of such explanations. Choice B is better but still understates the notion that most if not all crimes are committed by competent and rational individuals. Thus, choice B appears understated. Choice D is essentially valid but is both poorly conceptualized and vague in this context. In fact, the author does not actually address the issue of easy explanations here; rather, the point is that important alternative explanations most likely exist.

PASSAGE VII

43. **D** According to the passage, for most teenagers, learning to drive involves "peer pressure" as well as "parental dictates." To this extent, the author most accurately implies a struggle for independence from such forces and toward the assumed objectives behind learning to drive. Although choice A might look reasonable, the argument in the passage quite explicitly notes that rather than inevitably being connected to learning to be independent, learning to drive more often teaches the individual that he or she is, in fact, highly dependent. The young driver often assumes that driving and independence are concomitant; however, the author appears to argue quite the opposite. Choice B may also seem reasonable but is more likely an overstatement of the author's anxieties about driving. Alternatively, choice C appears to understate the dynamics involved in learning to drive.

44. **C** The liberating effects of driving appear most highly compromised by the demands of others restricting both access to vehicles and the purposes of driving. Note the author's references to being at the "mercy of . . . parents who owned the automobiles . . . [and] also the mercy of . . . friends who successively determined where . . . [to] go and what . . . [to] do." Although the author notes parental concerns over "fastidious" conduct on the road, competence appears more of a secondary concern for the author. Therefore, choice A can be eliminated. Choice B is inappropriate because the trials of instruction

more accurately lead to more independent driving and do eventually disappear from the experience. Choice C suffers from the same problems as choice A because it is more accurately described as a secondary concern.

45. **D** Considering the anxieties engendered in the individuals by "well-meaning" instructors and overseers, the best answer would be one that addressed either one or both of these dimensions of the passage. Therefore, choice D, which suggests a driver who is able to avoid at least some of these anxieties, is probably the best choice here. Choice A can be eliminated for two reasons: first, it is not really addressed by the author as a viable alternative; second, there is no basis for assuming that such challenges would necessarily be successful. Choice B may appear reasonable considering the author's admiration of such individuals; however, it does not allow the possibility that many drivers may well avoid the trials and tribulations that the author notes. Therefore, choice B fails to address the central issues here. Choice C suffers from the same problems as choice B in that it is more of an indirect consideration in the passage.

46. **A** Based on information in the passage, peer pressure is most accurately characterized as something that highly influences but need not necessarily consume or completely control the individual. As such, choice A appears to be the most appropriate answer. It is important to note here that although the author notes that peer demands upon teenagers appear completely unwarranted, there is no direct evaluation of these demands as necessarily unfair or destructive. Based on the previous observations, the assumption that peer pressure is necessarily unfair allows us to eliminate choice B. Although choice C appears reasonable, this observation says little about the actual characterization of peer pressure in the passage. Choice D is inappropriate because it characterizes peer pressure as all-consuming and the teenager as little more than under the control of peers. To this extent, choice D appears overstated considering information in the passage.

47. **D** Based on information in the passage, the biggest source of confusion for the author appears to be based on his observations about "where exactly [he] was located in [the] decision-making processes" concerning driving. Therefore, choice D appears to be the most appropriate answer because it addresses the actual role of the driver in the act of driving. Choice A points to the reasons behind having learned to drive, yet according to information in the passage the author appears to have been fully aware of the forces compelling him to learn to drive. Therefore, choice A appears to misunderstand the essence of the argument. Choice B suffers from the same problem because the author seems fully aware of the forces compelling Americans to learn to drive. Choice C may seem reasonable; however, it addresses simply the purposes of driving, and, once again, it seems as though the author quite simply saw his reasons for driving inextricably linked to the demands of others. Therefore, choice C can also be eliminated.

48. **B** The overwhelming number of cars in the United States has no clear bearing on the argument presented in the passage. However, it can be assumed that based on the logic of the passage, "the pressures to drive in this country are indeed overwhelming" for most teenagers and ultimately adult drivers. Therefore, choice B seems to be the most appropriate answer. Choice A suggests that Americans are seemingly unaware of the forces behind the need to drive and can, therefore, be eliminated. Choice C may be reasonable; however, the issues of overestimation simply are not addressed by the author in the passage. Indeed, most feel compelled to drive; however, this does not allow the reader to assume this is necessarily misdirected. Choice D is inappropriate because it bears no real connection to the question itself and, at best, reduces the argument to one based on individual psychopathology.

PASSAGE VIII

49. **B** Based on information in the passage, the general tone of the author appears to be one of qualified acceptance. The author notes his frustration with the political dynamics of allocating research and treatment dollars; however, he also notes that AIDS activism appears to be simply "playing the game" that any in search of funds must follow. The author does note that AIDS sufferers deserve compassion and scientific inquiry and even says that the successes of activists seem purely justified based on the realities of the "rough and tumble" of politics. Yet, he is also clearly concerned about the attention AIDS has received proportionate to that of other diseases. Although choice A might seem reasonable, the allowances made to AIDS activists and sufferers make this an inappropriate one. The author may seem frustrated but clearly is not indignant based on the information in the passage. Choice C can be eliminated for the same reasons; the author simply is not in opposition to such efforts. Choice D can also be eliminated because it appears to understate the author's frustration and skepticism regarding funding for treatment and research.

50. **D** As the passage indicates, the author feels that funding in general is relatively unsystematic. With respect to AIDS in particular, the author notes the centrality of "conspicuousness and constituency" and the high profile of those who suffer or have died of the disease. Although organization is also central to the success of those seeking funding, it is not offered in any of the choices. Choice A seems generally correct; however, the author cites it only as a general characteristic of funding decisions. Thus, although it is then a characteristic of AIDS funding, the particulars of this disease are not addressed by this observation. Choice B is easily eliminated in that the author notes that AIDS is only "now riding a crest of public support" and not one that is necessarily traditional. Choice C does appear relevant; however, no specific evidence is offered regarding AIDS itself and, thus, is offered only as a general characteristic of all government funding.

51. **B** In terms of the future of AIDS funding, the author makes concerted efforts to criticize the tactics of AIDS activists in terms of the need to consistently shift their approaches. Because the author's objective then seems to be the "unmasking" of what the author perceives as the weaknesses of each approach–particularly in terms of the extent of victimization–it seems reasonable to conclude that the author believes that public awareness of the epidemiology of the disease will eventually lead to the decline of public support. Choice A seems speculative in the absence of information to challenge the author's assertion that the disease is far more selective than advocates have suggested. It may be true, considering the changing characteristics of the disease; however, no such evidence is offered in the passage itself. Choice C can also be eliminated based on the author's assumption about the growing public awareness of the fallacies of the arguments offered by AIDS activists. Choice D also seems reasonable, yet once again, there is no evidence in the passage that increased competition is inevitably going to lead to the decline of AIDS funding.

52. **C** The author's discussion of phobia in paragraph three is used to illustrate not the justification for funding dollars but rather the tactics of the activists themselves. As the author notes, "the passion turns to a mere stridency when they take to the streets to protest a phobic society," and he calls attention to the loud and obtrusive quality of the activism. Choice A seems logically connected but is not in this passage. The author does, in fact, discuss accusations of phobia in a relatively negative light and, thus, fails to address more fundamental issues of discrimination and hostility. Choice B has little to do with the argument itself and is, in fact, countered by the author's observations that funding for AIDS appears to be enjoying a relatively high level of public support. Choice D can be eliminated based on the author's observations that the passion is transformed as activists take to the streets.

53. **C** Choice A can be eliminated based on the fact that the author does not necessarily suggest that diseases acquired through intentional acts deserve less attention. He is only frustrated by public campaigns that apparently mislead the public on the facts. Choice B suffers from similar problems in that it makes the same assumptions in terms of efforts to set funding priorities. Choice D is logically eliminated.

54. **C** Based on this passage, the author believes funding for the treatment and research of any disease needs reevaluation. Although the author provides no specific details on funding procedures, this criterion needs to be carefully reconsidered because AIDS funding has relied heavily on the notoriety of victims of AIDS. Based on the objections raised by the author, the characteristics of the populations should be considerations in the allocation of research and treatment dollars. At the very least, these characteristics should be made clear to the general public, and the author indirectly suggests that they do matter. Therefore, choice A can be eliminated. Choice B may seem reasonable; however,

there is little information provided in the passage to support this. Choice D is one of the bases cited by the author in his examination of AIDS funding and, thus, needs to be more cautiously considered.

55. **D** The author's reference to "rough justice" clearly is connected to congressional interest in diseases. Thus, the author's objective appears to be that of drawing attention to some equitableness in the allocation of federal funds because members of Congress are human beings and will inevitably "experience most of the medical tragedies that life has to offer." Although choice A obviously is connected to this central theme, the more important point appears to be the result of this human vulnerability rather than the vulnerability itself. This vulnerability seemingly provides for some ultimate form of justice. Choice A, as noted, is obviously connected but is not the central point of the author's observation. The more important point is that tragedy leads to support for particular diseases, and choice A is a rather secondary concern of the passage. Choice B can be eliminated considering the author's seeming acceptance of the realities of the funding process, despite his frustration. Choice C has the same weakness.

56. **B** There seems little doubt that the central objective of the author is to demonstrate the importance of political strategies to successfully gain public support and funding for treatment and research of any disease. This point is supported by the author's critique of the AIDS campaigns as well as his critique of the political dimensions of providing support. Although choice A may seem obvious, there is clearly a greater objective implied by the author here. The critique of the AIDS campaign is invariably connected to larger concerns with funding, as supported by the author's more general attack on the "archaic, chaotic, and almost random" nature of the process itself. Choice C is eliminated easily because the author makes no such reference to the need for AIDS patients to bear the burden of research and treatment alone; remember that the author is sympathetic with the campaign. Choice D seems reasonable; however, the neglect of other diseases seems less the objective here because the author does not come out necessarily in favor of any particular interest. Other diseases are noted only as bases of comparison rather than in terms of their favoritism for funding.

PASSAGE IX

57. **C** As the author notes, standard drug definitions technically include everything that affects, by its chemical or physical nature, the living organism. As such, the definition includes not only those things traditionally considered nondrugs but also a wide range of activities. Therefore, standard pharmacological definitions are clearly assumed to be overly inclusive; they include far more than necessarily intended and scientifically appropriate. Choice A is inappropriate because it may challenge standard scientific definitions, but it does not render

them formally invalid. The author notes that standard drug definitions do indeed claim to be objective based on scientific research; however, this claim is challenged in the passage. Choice B is inappropriate because it has little bearing on the actual classification of drugs because science does indeed have the ability to note drug effects. Choice D can be eliminated because such an acknowledgment is necessarily relevant in the challenge to pharmacological classification.

58. **D** Despite the author's disillusionment with standard drug classification, there is little justification offered in the passage for any choice other than D. The author offers no argument that scientific reasoning is necessarily sparse, faulty, or illogical. The central point of the passage is that standard scientific knowledge is misguided in that it assumes the purely objective nature of its conclusions represents a complete and exclusive explanation of what drugs are and what exactly they do. Choice A suggests that the scientific category is essentially meaningless; however, such an observation seems to overlook the author's observation that it has great meaning in terms of its consequences for how certain individuals actually define drugs. Thus, choice A can be eliminated.

59. **C** As the information in the passage notes, the author's major objection to standard pharmacological definitions is precisely that they fail to exclude those properties that are alien nondrug substances. As such, the author seems to conclude that the scientific category of drugs is effectively nonexclusive. There is no doubt that the scientific category of drugs is, in fact, extremely meaningful if not extremely powerful. However, the point of the passage is that the author wishes to challenge whether the category is necessarily a valid one. Therefore, choice A is inappropriate. Choice B is easily eliminated on the same terms—the category genuinely exists; however, it is questionable. Choice D also is eliminated easily in that it is clearly based on scientific research.

60. **D** Of all of the claims listed here, the most weakly supported appears to be choice D. The author simply notes in the passage that different definitions exist and cites that "[a] policeman . . . will think of drugs in primarily legal terms: substances whose possession is against the law." Beyond this, little information is offered to support this particular example. Choice A is, in fact, the central point of the passage and is made relevant by the majority of observations made by the author. Choice B is also central to the author's argument as shown by numerous examples. Choice C appears just as well supported.

61. **D** Considering the information in the passage, it would seem clear that the author is relatively skeptical about the distinction between illicit and licit drugs. The central argument appears to be that such distinctions are based purely on the decisions of human beings. Note the observation that "the category 'drug' is humanly fabricated . . . [w]hat is or is not a drug is decided not by nature, but by us, by humans—by definition." Choice A may seem reasonable; however, it seems too sweeping even in this context. There is no evidence in the passage

that the author wishes to eliminate all sanctions against the use of drugs; rather, he suggests a reevaluation of existing categories. Choice B is also inappropriate to the extent that the existing distinction between illicit and licit drugs is actually quite meaningful; however, it is not necessarily valid. Choice C can be questioned on the same basis as is choice A in that such a relaxation will necessarily address the central issues with which he is concerned.

62. **A** Considering current legislation calling for the legalization of marijuana for medicinal purposes, the author would be most likely to lend support simply because of his feelings about the ambiguity of existing scientific research. As the author notes throughout the passage, existing pharmacological definitions do not unambiguously define all such substances. Choice B is inappropriate because it is clear from the passage that the categorization of marijuana as illegal is well founded in the decisions of, at the very least, legal authorities, despite the implied ambiguity of scientific work. Choice C has the same problems as choice B because it fails to address the politics of classification. Choice D, although potentially true, is easily eliminated simply because such issues are not addressed in the passage.

63. **A** Considering the logic of the passage, the observation that would most strongly support the general theme of the passage would be that which emphasized some example of the ambiguity and inconsistency of drug legislation itself. As such, the observation about the important legal distinction between morphine and heroin appears to be the most supportive. Choice B may be true; however, its bearing on the central concern of the passage is relatively negligible because it is simply an observation that a legal "drug" is highly destructive. Importantly, the author wishes to note that substances are categorized rather arbitrarily. To this extent, cigarettes do provide a good example of legal "destruction"; however, this example is less effective in establishing the distinction than choice A. Choice C is essentially true; however, both are illegal and are less effective in making the author's point. Choice D is also true but seems irrelevant here.

64. **C** As the passage implies, reference to "drug abuse" is considered by the author to be relatively value-laden because the definitions of drugs themselves are based on the definition of subjectively motivated human beings. Thus, choice C is the most appropriate selection. Choice A is eliminated easily on the basis of the author's observations that the label of "addiction" seems relatively value-laden as well. Logically, according to the passage, the "reality" of addiction is just as arbitrary as the classification of the drug involved. Choice B is also inappropriate considering the selectivity of psychoactive drugs by the particular individuals as the genuinely acceptable basis for defining drugs. Choice D may seem reasonable; however, the subjective definition of the drug user, considering the logic of the passage, would be based entirely on the definitions available—particularly those suggesting the fallibility of the user.

65. **C** As the author notes, we should search "outside the substances themselves, to see how they are defined, used, and conceptualized." In combination with other information in the passage, the author implies that the intrinsic properties of drugs tell us little in terms of developing some form of reasonable classification. Thus, the central point is that the variability of intrinsic properties makes the establishment of an objective category relatively impossible. Choice A is inappropriate because the establishment of such properties is relatively well-founded, yet it still tells us little for the purposes of general classification. Choice B has the same problems in that first, it is not necessarily true, and second, it offers little in terms of classification. Choice D is logically eliminated.

VERBAL REASONING PRACTICE TEST 3

Suggested Time: 85 minutes

Directions: There are nine reading passages in the Verbal Reasoning test. Each passage is followed by several questions. After reading a passage, select one best answer to each question. If you are not certain of an answer, eliminate the alternatives that you know to be incorrect, and then select an answer from the remaining alternatives.

Passage I (Questions 1–7)

The accomplishments of democracy in America have been well chronicled by innumerable authors. At the same time, however, one should note that "democracy in America" has its critics as well, and the problems of the American experiment are indeed just as well documented. Robert Bellah notes that as early as the 1830s, Alexis de Tocqueville noticed certain features of American life that he believed endangered traditional relationships, whether of kinship, religion, or civic friendship. Tocqueville wrote: "Democracy does not create strong attachments between man and man, but it does put their ordinary relations on an easier footing." Tocqueville's argument was that in older societies, one knew where one stood relative to others because of the existence of a network of established statutes and roles, each of which implied an appropriate form of attachment. In the mobile and egalitarian society of the United States, people could meet more easily and their interaction was more open, but the ties between them were more likely to be casual and transient. A further reason for this casualness and transience has to do with what Tocqueville calls the American's "restlessness in the midst of prosperity." He says, "In America, I have seen the freest and best educated of men in circumstances the happiest to be found in the world; yet it seemed to me that a cloud habitually hung on their brow, and they seemed serious and almost sad even in their pleasures," because they "never stop thinking of the good things they have not got." This restlessness and sadness in pursuit of the good life is intensified, says Tocqueville, by "the competition of all," which in the United States replaces the aristocratic privilege of some. So the efforts and enjoyments of Americans are livelier than in traditional societies, but the disappointments of their hopes and desires are keener, and their "minds are more anxious and on edge." How could such restless, competitive, and anxious people sustain such enduring relationships, when "they clutch everything and hold nothing fast?"

In his early declarations, Tocqueville appeared a soothsayer. George M. Beard's *American Nervousness* later popularized the term *neurasthenia,* a generalized malaise that seemed to be affecting large numbers of "civilized, refined, and educated" Americans at that time. Although Beard and others blamed the new national disease on such heterogeneous phenomena as railway travel and the telegraph, overwork and more specialized occupations, rapid turnover of ideas, and so forth, they tended to sum up its causes under the phrase "modern civilization." Nervous exhaustion is "developed, fostered, and perpetuated with the progress of civilization, and the advance of culture and refinement, and . . . it is oftener met with in cities than in the country, is more marked and more frequent at the desk, the pulpit, and in the counting room than in the shop or on the farm." Thus, Beard was as much taking pride in this modern affliction that affected only the "most evolutionarily advanced" as he was deploring its causes.

Reflecting on this "outbreak," Bellah notes that this first massive awakening of the concern of Americans for their mental health allows us to make out a key change in the nature of interpersonal relationships. Beard himself points to "the liberty allowed, and the stimulus given, to Americans to rise out of the position in which they were born, whatever that may be, and to aspire to the highest possibilities of fortune and glory" as a force in producing American nervousness, along with the fact that "in all classes there is a constant friction and unrest—a painful striving to see who shall be the highest."

In establishing the larger social–structural context, Bellah notes as well that the period preoccupied with "American nervousness" was also the period in which a national market was depriving the small towns and regional cities of their effective independence and throwing increasing numbers of Americans into a national occupational world based on education, mobility, and the ability to compete. Unfortunately, what this great social transformation meant for individuals was that they faced challenges and uncertainties for which they were not prepared.

Adapted from Robert N. Bellah, *Habits of the Heart*. © 1995 by Robert N. Bellah.

1. Which of the following observations best captures the central point of the passage?

A. Americans are far more nervous than the citizens of other countries.
B. The historical experience of Americans has made them far more nervous than the citizens of other countries.
C. The democratic tradition of the United States has obvious negative consequences.
D. The democratic tradition of the United States has been complicated by technological advances.

2. According to the author of the passage, what has been the greatest source of "neurasthenia" historically?

A. The rapid progress of technology in general
B. The inability to deal with the rapid progress of technology
C. The failure to deal with the rapid progress of technology
D. The changing context of American politics

3. The discussion of American "preoccupation" with nervousness suggests that:

A. most Americans fail to understand the consequences of life in this country.
B. few Americans understand the consequences of advancing technology.
C. the legacy of the American experience will always contribute to restlessness in this country.
D. prosperity can be both advantageous and disadvantageous.

4. The author's observations that "Beard was as much taking pride in this modern affliction that affected the 'most evolutionarily advanced' as he was deploring its causes" appear to mean that:

A. Beard was rather uncertain about the actual effects of advancing technology on the American public.
B. Beard's explanation is essentially elitist in character.
C. the poor in America were being spared this fundamental tension in American life.
D. all of the above.

5. Considering the central message of the passage, the author would most likely be in agreement with which of the following contemporary observations about life in America?

   A. The United States continues to be one of the most consumer-oriented nations in the world, but it is also characterized by relatively low levels of political participation.
   B. Americans are currently experiencing a "back-to-basics" orientation and eschewing the material aspects of life.
   C. The historical experience of the United States has contributed greatly to a decline in the standard of living in this country.
   D. Most Americans are likely to experience some form of mental illness at some point in their lives.

6. Based on information in the passage, Beard's description of a "class system" in the United States is perhaps best described as:

   A. unique in comparison to most other western, developed nations.
   B. virtually nonexistent.
   C. inconsequential in terms of dictating the terms of political participation.
   D. inconsequential in terms of experiencing the effects of advancing technology.

7. Restlessness, as described in the passage, can best be equated with which of the following ideas?

   A. Some fundamental dissatisfaction with the new social and political demands facing most Americans
   B. Disillusionment with early political experiences in the United States
   C. The inexperience of early American political figures
   D. None of the above

Passage II (Questions 8–15)

Despite her overwhelming popularity, Madonna has her adversaries. One such adversary, Joseph Sobran, challenges the singer on purely technical grounds. Sobran admits that Madonna is a genius at getting attention. In fact, he argues that everything she does gets attention—her records, videos, movies, and relationships. When she showed up at the Cannes Film Festival with her hair dyed a different color, her face appeared on the front page of the New York *Daily News*. She has been on the cover of every magazine except *National Geographic*.

But Sobran asks critically, "How does she do it?" On more than one occasion, Madonna has freely admitted in an interview that she's not a great singer, dancer, or even—at least in repose—a great looker. She also admitted to having average acting skills. Yet, she has the most flamboyantly theatrical personality since . . . well, who was the last one? Bette Davis? Joan Crawford? Some people have what I can only call contagious vanity. You may even dislike them, but you cannot take your eyes off them. Madonna is like that. In a country where people want to be liked, she dares you to hate her.

Sobran does look to the provocative Camille Paglia, herself a sort of antifeminist feminist, as a singular source of support for the singer. Paglia notes that "Madonna exposes the puritanism and suffocating ideology of American feminism. Madonna has taught young women to be fully female and sexual while still exercising total control over their lives. She shows girls how to be attractive, sensual, energetic, ambitious, aggressive, and funny—all at the same time."

So Sobran will admit that she's undeniably magnetic, but it's a calculating magnetism, a carefully constructed aura of kink and danger. If she seems to be shattering conventions, she's also there to pick up the pieces. One of her videos shows her in a Catholic Church adoring a statue of a saint who comes to life and kisses her passionately. She receives the stigmata, and there are burning crosses and things, and . . . well, again, you get the idea: a deliberate fusion of such themes as sex, race, and religion. These elements are combined in surreal montage, and the effect is eerie and shocking.

An even more provocative video did succeed in upsetting people, and even easygoing music video stations refused to play it. "The video is pornographic," Paglia writes. "It's decadent. And it's fabulous. The music video television station was right to ban it." But she chides Madonna for copping out on an evening television news show by pleading "her love of children and her social activism." If you want to shock people, go ahead and shock them. But don't blame them for being shocked.

But the key for Sobran is the trouble with Madonna—that she wants to have it both ways. Indeed, he notes that one problem in writing about her is that everything sounds like a double entendre. She clearly knows what she's doing, but wants to pretend she doesn't.

In a recent magazine interview Madonna gets defensive: "People will say, 'She knows the camera is on, she's just acting.' But even if I am acting, there's a truth in my acting. You could watch it and say, 'I still don't know Madonna,' and good. Because you will never know the real me. Ever." You mean there is more?

But one wonders if, in fact, Sobran actually cares to pursue this line of inquiry. He states that if we never know the real Madonna, we will not have Madonna to blame for it. She talks about herself incessantly; she poses for photo stills dressed up as Marilyn Monroe and other sexpots. It's as if her privacy might unfairly deprive us of something. Or rather, as if she wanted to become all the fascinating women of the past, and reveal their mysteries to us. Instead, she creates the disconcerting impression that all the mystery may have been bogus; maybe those women *were* like her: self-absorbed, uninteresting people who talked in clichés about "art" and "truth" when they were not talking about themselves. One would rather not know.

Adapted from Joseph Sobran, "Madonna is a Vapid Pop Figure" in *Culture Wars*. © 1991 by Greenhaven Press.

8. Based on the tone of the passage, which of the following statements best describes the author's attitude toward Madonna as an entertainer?

A. Madonna essentially demonstrates little or no creative talent whatsoever.
B. Madonna's creative talent is only secondary to her abilities to shock the American public.
C. Madonna's creative talents are significant, but they are subsumed by her need for public attention.
D. Madonna's creative talents would be better demonstrated by using a more conventional approach to entertainment in general.

9. Considering the commentary on Madonna's religious dimensions, it would seem reasonable to suggest that:

A. Madonna is best described as a religious heretic.
B. Madonna appears to profoundly misunderstand the tenets of Catholicism.
C. Madonna's apparent license with religious imagery appears profoundly antireligious.
D. Madonna's manipulation of religious imagery indicates a deeply disturbed young woman.

10. When the author notes that "if we never know the real Madonna, we will not have Madonna to blame for it," he appears to mean that:

A. her efforts at being provocative have, in fact, been dismal failures.
B. the entertainer makes empty efforts to proclaim her privacy despite her high public profile.
C. her public admissions that she is misunderstood remain rather empty apologies.
D. Madonna's private life is, in fact, highly public.

11. Considering the stance taken in the passage on the entertainer's publicity tactics, which of the following statements would probably best describe the appetites of the consuming public in the United States?

A. Americans are rather unsophisticated in terms of judging the merits of contemporary entertainers.
B. Americans appear more concerned with the image of entertainers and unconcerned with the actual talent of the individual.
C. Americans are easily distracted by showmanship.
D. Americans are just as often attracted by the magnetism of entertainers as they are by the talent of the individual.

12. Based on information presented in the passage, which statement best points to Madonna's showmanship?

A. The progressive character of Madonna's sexual imagery
B. The entertainer's denial of feminism
C. The nonsexual nature of Madonna's imagery
D. The ability of a relatively untalented woman to achieve such a high level of success

13. When the author parallels Madonna with other figures in the entertainment industry, his objective is best described as which of the following statements?

A. To demonstrate the prevalence of personal vanity in the entertainment industry
B. To draw a clearer distinction between apparently talented and untalented entertainers
C. To suggest that most Americans have an inappropriate need to be admired or liked in general
D. To demonstrate that most of the fascinating women of the past have been largely superficial and self-absorbed

14. In terms of the logic of the passage, the American press is best characterized by the author as:

A. contributing to the decadence of American society.
B. blatantly irresponsible in their contributions to Madonna's success.
C. simply mirroring the tastes of the American public.
D. just as unsophisticated as the average American.

15. The message conveyed by the passage suggests that:

A. Madonna is an extremely liberated woman.
B. Madonna is no more aware of what she represents than is anyone else.
C. Madonna is fully unaware of what she is doing as a public figure.
D. Madonna's public image is highly ambiguous.

Passage III (Questions 16–21)

Progress in all fields of technology—medical, social, pure and applied sciences, and in engineering—would be impossible without the objective exchange of information. For example, the progress in a technical man's profession is blocked when he is unable to present technical facts. To be of use, the work of a scientist or engineer must be recorded so that others can understand, and often the written record is all that remains as testimony of the work after the experimental and testing structures have been disassembled. The written record is the end product, the enduring proof that something has been uncovered and offered for the use of society.

If the result of a man's work cannot be expressed clearly, it cannot be used effectively, and the value of a man is judged accordingly. From his written reports, other men infer the qualities of his mind and the order of his method. The ability to state facts clearly and accurately, organize a variety of elements into a unified structure, derive logical conclusions from a host of disparate facts, and convey information in an intelligible language wins instant respect and opens avenues of opportunity for professional progress. If the sentences and words are precise and meaningful, the reasoning sound, the planning logical, then the alert director or supervisor can see the merits of the research, testing, and the work itself.

But if the reasoning is muddled or slanted, the supervisor will guess that the writer is trying to hide inadequacies; if the planning is haphazard, he will assume the writer's logic is weak; and if the language is esoteric or spotted with jargon, the alert supervisor will imagine the writer has little creativity and is trying to cover this gaping hole with a curtain of learning.

Students should realize at the outset that writing is a craft to be mastered rather than a science to be learned. Though rules of the craft are iterated in a variety of texts, and examples are offered by our finest authors, mastery can be obtained only through the writing experience. Employing the rules and the examples in his own trials and errors, the technical man develops the most important facility for writing—a critical sense. It tells him when the writing is obscure, illogical, or awkward. And as the sense develops, he learns to do the things that change a poor presentation into an effective one.

The critical sense he develops also has a direct bearing on his laboratory work. To write effectively, the author must take time to review what he has accomplished. If the work cannot be communicated logically, then the material itself may not be clear enough to the writer. Reexamination often reveals obscurities, inaccuracies, inconsistencies, and perhaps deeper problems that should have been attacked before the reporter proceeded to his conclusions. The act of organizing the work for communication assures a critical view of the whole and serves as a check on its validity and value.

The common denominator between the craft of writing and the method of science is logic. There are skills to be mastered as in other aspects of any technological field, but the technical writer has already been trained in some discipline; already he has formed the habit of logical thinking. Writing is an extension and new application of this habit.

Adapted from Lawrence Heftel, *The Craft of Technical Writing*. © 1996 by University Press.

16. When the author notes that technological progress would be impossible without the objective exchange of information, he is suggesting that:

A. subjectivity has no place in the medical, social, pure, and applied sciences.
B. subjectivity has been a major obstacle to the advance of all sciences.
C. subjectivity compromises the integrity of scientific work.
D. subjectivity compromises the exchange of scientific information.

17. Which of the following observations best describes the author's central objective in the passage? Scientific writing:

A. should strive first and foremost for clarity.
B. is all too often characterized by poor expression.
C. should strive first and foremost to gain respect from peers.
D. is all too often characterized by efforts to mask poor research.

18. According to information in the passage, the relationship between a scientist's critical sense and the quality of his professional work can best be understood as:

A. complementary.
B. reciprocal.
C. superficial.
D. obscure.

19. The most effective scientific writer is the individual who is able to:

A. recognize the limitations of his own expertise.
B. acknowledge the consequences of poor scientific presentation.
C. use the writing process in the conduct of sound scientific research in general.
D. change a poor presentation into an effective one.

20. Which of the following observations best captures the attitude expressed in the passage toward the use of scientific jargon in scientific research? Scientific jargon:

A. is little more than esoteric.
B. is all too commonplace in scientific writing.
C. can substitute for sound scientific research.
D. frequently is used to mask poor scientific research.

21. The observation that "the written record is the enduring proof that something has been uncovered and offered for the use of society" is carefully based on:

A. the understanding that the author has been sufficiently trained in the habit of logical thinking.
B. the expectation that the written record sufficiently demonstrates the merits of the research.
C. the belief that merits of the research have been appropriately recorded.
D. all of the above.

Passage IV (Questions 22–28)

In an effort to offer some interesting commentary on contemporary nationalism, Robert Blakely has taken it upon himself to warn Americans of an impending crisis to the north. As he notes, nations, like stars, burn out. Amid the world's constellations of 180 or so countries, some, such as Austria or Greece, supernovas in their day, have seen their once brilliant empires and cultures dim or go dark, leaving their mother nations lusterless bit players on the international stage. Others, brief comets of glory or conquest, have flamed out, becoming forgotten epochs or black holes of social and political chaos, civilizations in abandon.

Chastising Americans for their preoccupation with the Soviet Union, half a world away and itself torn apart, Blakely argues that Americans were transfixed by the drama, although we shared little with the Russians this past half century other than nuclear masterdom and the dread of mutual annihilation. Yet across our northern border, Canada—most of whose 28 million people share with us the same language, democratic ideals, and a galaxy of commercial enterprises—also faces the prospect of dissolution. North America's once dismissable attic of the inconsequential—now our primary trading partner and strategic shield against still formidable nuclear forces—could splinter into two or more states before the century's end. And Americans seem largely indifferent to, or unaware of, the consequences.

Yet the crisis to the north is nothing new, and Canadians have been questioning the survivability of their country since its birth about 90 years after the Declaration of Independence. In the 1990s, the question has become painfully acute: Will Canada still exist as a country at the end of the decade, or will it have disintegrated, a victim of the tensions of its troubled past and present? Nearly half of Canada's populace, when polled a while back, answered "yes" to the second part of the question.

Locating the source of the problem, Blakely points largely to the gaping wound of Quebec's disaffection. Its French-speaking majority has for more than two centuries agitated for English Canada to recognize the province and its status for what most Québecois in their souls fervently believe: Quebec, in all but the formalities, is already a separate nation. Now, finally spurred by the sulfurous defiance of Quebec's separatists and the sense of betrayal among English Canadians, Canada's two founding peoples, hunkered in their separate quarters under the same roof, seem bent on dissolving their marriage.

Our image of Canada has thus been sadly superficial, and while outwardly civil to one another, our neighbors have managed until now to submerge their differences in the interests of serving each other's needs: English Canada's for retaining a vibrant francophone culture within the nation to lend it greater distinctiveness; Quebec's for staying allied to a strong and supportive national economy. But as for that economy, hobbled by debts and systemic failings, it has in the early 1990s faltered through recession and a shaky recovery. Quebecers have turned further away from the rest of Canada. Forever sure of their cultural superiority, they now feel confident enough to oversee their economic destiny as well.

Thus, we have long misunderstood Canada, and most Americans comfortably assume that Canadians are too decent, too passive a people to propel themselves into such a breakup. The world has been suckered by such assumptions for much of the century. A more realistic view is that Canadians, surfeited by their antagonisms and stymied in resolving them, might let their nation sunder by default. If that happens, they, we, and the rest of the world will share painful costs. Gone for Canadians would be much of the economic reward of their union, their hard-won international stature, and their enviable tradition of civility. For the United States and the rest of the world, the stakes encompass the fate of Canada as our biggest partner by far in trade and finance, our closest NATO ally, and a reliable force for good in international councils around the globe.

Adapted from Robert Blakely, *Breakup*. © 1994 by Spencer Press.

22. Based on information in the passage, the historical ambivalence of Americans toward Canada is best described as:

A. a misunderstanding of the importance of Canada as a trading partner and strategic shield against still formidable nuclear forces.
B. the result of Canada's relatively inconsequential historical importance on the world stage.
C. a lack of awareness of the threat of Quebec separatism.
D. the result of a preoccupation with other more formidable political opponents.

23. From the reasoning presented in the passage, the author would be most likely to support which of the following United States political stances toward Canada?

A. A more aggressive American effort to force the Province of Quebec to remain part of the Canadian Union
B. The promotion of more aggressive collective American–Canadian efforts to establish French as an official North American language
C. A more concerted American effort to recognize North American political struggles in general
D. A more general American preparation for the political consequences of the separation of Quebec

24. According to the passage, the contemporary discontent in Quebec appears to be largely based on:

A. the feeling that Quebecers are culturally superior.
B. the failure of the Canadian government to recognize a vibrant francophone culture.
C. the unshakable belief that Quebec is already a separate nation.
D. none of the above.

25. Considering the tone of the passage, it seems apparent that most Canadians are skeptical about the future of their nation because of:

A. historical experience of the country.
B. the failure of the Canadian economy to recover from debts and systematic failings.
C. a lack of commitment to continuation by both English and French Canadians.
D. the potential of the Canadian government to reconcile the interests of the French.

26. The author's opening statements about nationhood in general suggest that:

A. Canada is seemingly doomed to dissolution.
B. nationhood itself must be based on sound political footings.
C. nationhood is a relatively precarious existence.
D. civilization and nationhood are not necessarily one and the same.

27. The characterization of the political sympathies of most Canadians is best described by which of the following statements? Most Canadians:

A. are willing to surrender their national identity because of a profound disillusionment.
B. appear relatively ambivalent toward their own nationhood.
C. are clearly fearful about their prospects for continuation as a nation.
D. are at best cautiously optimistic about the prospects of continued nationhood.

28. When the author observes that the dissolution of Canada may bring with it the destruction of "a reliable force for good in international councils around the globe," he is most likely referring to:

A. the importance of Canada's historical efforts at the reconciliation of different cultures.
B. the loss of an important political ally of the United States.
C. the importance of the political neutrality historically demonstrated by Canada.
D. all of the above.

Passage V (Questions 29–35)

Although nomadism is a more primitive state than agriculturalism, it is scarcely less specialized, and in the medieval period nomad societies often possessed a culture comparable in level of attainment to that in the contemporary settled communities. Flocks of sheep, goats, and horses provide all the raw materials necessary for a simple life and a good many luxuries too. Indeed, the nomad often exceeded the agriculturist in wealth because if his pasture was poor in quality, it was nearly limitless in extent, and while he could keep moving, his herds could be of great size.

The ability to move far and fast was the keynote of the nomad's existence and the root of his success in war. Napoleon's dictum of military "momentum" states that the real strength of an army is the product of its size and speed. Nomad armies, in which every man was not only horsed but had a spare mount in tow, could move at a speed that for the era was phenomenal. Because of this mobility, they gave a totally misleading impression of enormous numbers, and the word horde, originally a term for a Turko-Mongol regiment, came to mean an innumerable swarm. This erroneous impression was strengthened by the nomads' locust-like capacity for thorough destruction, which stemmed partly from the harshness of steppe and desert life, partly from their compelling hate and fear of the ever-multiplying peasants. Terror spread before a nomad advance and did much to prepare the way for victory.

There is another analogy with locusts that is worth pursuing. Locusts usually live out their lives as solitary grasshoppers in the areas of scrub that are scattered through the desert. A succession of good years causes an enlargement of the scrub islands and, consequently, of the locust population. If the next year is catastrophically bad, the islands shrink to a fraction of their original size, and the locusts are crowded together. The sight of hundreds of others of its kind, milling about in front of it, stimulates the locust to metamorphose. When the change to the migratory form is complete, the whole swarm rises in a cloud from the island they have eaten bare and sets out for pastures new.

How big a part such purely climatic causes played in initiating nomadic movements is debatable. Attempts have been made to relate the history of Asiatic movement to a cyclical desiccation of the continent, but probably the mechanism of explosive migration is much too sensitive to be a guide to long-term fluctuations. It is obvious, however, that physical factors of this type were responsible for much of the unrest that at times took hold of the nomadic world and that is usually described in purely political terms.

Of the four great nomadic nations, the Arabs, Berbers, Turks, and Mongols, the first two have histories that are part of the greater story of Islam. Their successes led them to give up nomadism and settle on the lands they had conquered, and though occasionally new tribes (Murabits, Qarmatians) swept from the desert to overthrow the Empires established by their forebears, there was never any attempt to impose the desert way of life on the settled communities of the Near-East area. The Turks and Mongols were far more intolerant and nearly always ignored the habits of the populations of which they made themselves masters.

Adapted from Peter Davidson, *The Atlas of Medieval History*. © 1991 by Historical Book Publishing.

29. According to information in the passage, nomad societies have been misunderstood largely because:

A. they have all too often been contrasted with contemporary settled communities.
B. they have historically been considered primitive.
C. of our failure to understand the dynamics of nomadic existence.
D. of a misleading impression of enormous numbers.

30. The reference to Napoleonic military strategy is used in the passage to best illustrate:

A. the military sophistication of nomad armies.
B. the importance of instilling terror in the minds of potential combatants.
C. a contrast of nomad armies with the military expertise of more settled communities.
D. the military expedience of nomad armies.

31. Based on the logic of the passage, the author would most likely argue that the major impediment to the material success of early settled communities versus nomad communities was the:

A. failure of settled communities to mount a successful military defense.
B. inability of settled communities to relocate when necessary.
C. environmental constraints faced by settled communities.
D. potential wealth of settled communities.

32. The parallel drawn between nomad communities and locusts is used by the author to argue that:

A. migration was a central feature of all nomad societies.
B. nomad societies were largely characterized by collectives of relatively solitary individuals.
C. nomad societies were highly adaptive collectives.
D. the pressures faced by nomad societies were exclusively dependent on environmental conditions.

33. Considering the intellectual controversies discussed in the passage, it seems reasonable to assume that, with respect to the movement of nomad communities, the author believes that:

A. scholars, in fact, understand very little about the dynamics of nomadic life.
B. climatic causes probably played a relatively negligible role.
C. explosive migration is far too sporadic to allow for explanation.
D. climatic causes can provide only a partial explanation.

34. The fact that only two of the great nomadic nations were led to abandon nomadism is explained by the author as the result of:

A. the successful conquering of settled communities.
B. their tolerance and acceptance of the habits of conquered communities.
C. their abilities to abandon the nomadic lifestyle and adapt to settled ways of life.
D. none of the above.

35. Which of the following statements would best describe the more contemporary relevance of this passage? The success of any community is highly dependent on its ability to:

A. adapt to changing political conditions.
B. utilize completely and effectively the resources at its disposal.
C. adapt to changing environmental conditions.
D. represent itself as more formidable than it may actually be.

Passage VI (Questions 36–42)

Despite the preponderance of popular tales of early explorers, no one knows who the first European visitors to the New World were. Credit usually goes to the Vikings, who reached the New World in approximately AD 1000, but others could have been there earlier. An ancient Latin text, the *Navitagio Sancti Brendani Abbatis*, or *The Voyage of St. Brendan the Abbot*, recounts with persuasive detail a 7-year trip to a land across the sea claimed to have been made by this Irish saint and a band of acolytes some four centuries before the Vikings—and this, it was said, on the advice of another Irishman who claimed to have been there earlier still.

In fact, Bill Bryson argues that even the Vikings did not think themselves the first. Their sagas record that when they first arrived in the New World they were chased from the beach by a group of wild white people. They subsequently heard from natives of a settlement of Caucasians who "wore white garments and . . . carried poles before them to which rags were attached"—precisely how an Irish religious procession might have looked to the uninitiated. Whether by Irish or Vikings—or Italians or Bretons or any of the other many groups for whom credit has been sought—crossing the Atlantic in the Middle Ages was not quite as daring a feat as it would first appear, even allowing for the fact that it was done in small, open boats. The North Atlantic is conveniently scattered with islands that could serve as stepping-stones (e.g., the Shetland Islands, the Faeroes, Iceland, Greenland, Baffin Island). It would be more possible to sail from Scandinavia to Canada without once crossing more than 250 miles of open sea.

Bryson notes that if we can be sure of anything it is that Greenland—and thus, technically, North America—was discovered in AD 982 by Eric the Red, father of Leif Ericsson (or Leif Eiriksson), and that he and his followers began settling it in AD 986. Anyone who has ever flown over the frozen wastes of Greenland could be excused for wondering what they saw in the place. The most natural thing would be to head west to see what was out there. In approximately AD 1000, according to the sagas, Leif Ericsson did just that. His expedition discovered a new landmass, probably Baffin Island, far up in northern Canada, over a thousand miles north of the present-day United States, and many other places, most notably the region they called Vinland.

Yet, what is perhaps most interesting is that Vinland's location is a tantalizing historical puzzle. Through careful readings of the sagas and calculations of Viking sailing times, various scholars have put Vinland all over the place—on Newfoundland or Nova Scotia, in Massachusetts, even as far south as Virginia. The name is no help. According to the sagas, the Vikings called it Vinland because of the grapevines they found growing in profusion there. One possible explanation is that Vinland was a mistranslation. Vinber, the Viking word for grapes, could be used to describe many other fruits—cranberries, gooseberries, and red currants among them—that might have been found at these northern latitudes. Another possibility is that Vinland was merely a bit of deft propaganda designed to encourage settlement. These were, after all, the people who thought up the name Greenland.

Adapted from Bill Bryson, *Made In America*.

36. Which of the following statements best represents the central theme of the passage?

A. The history of the Vikings is largely misunderstood.
B. The Vikings' claim to have been the first visitors to the New World is unfounded.
C. The history of the Vikings is shrouded in propaganda.
D. There are important aspects of New World history that remain unclear.

37. According to information in the passage, the first "recorded" visit to the New World occurred approximately:

A. AD 986.
B. AD 600.
C. AD 982.
D. AD 1000.

38. Which of the following statements best describes the tone found throughout the passage?

A. A critical stance toward existing historical knowledge
B. A sarcastic stance toward existing historical knowledge
C. A skeptical stance toward existing historical knowledge
D. A humorous stance toward existing historical knowledge

39. Based on information in the passage, it could be argued that the author is perhaps most compelled by which of the following popular misconceptions about New World history?

A. People tend to assume that Vinland's location is relatively easy to pinpoint.
B. People tend to assume that ocean crossings are relatively overwhelming feats.
C. Most people believe the Vikings were relatively sophisticated early explorers.
D. Most people believe Europeans discovered the New World.

40. In the author's discussion of Vinland, which of the following statements best describes his general conclusion?

A. The region of Vinland most likely never existed.
B. The region of Vinland is best described as the product of lively historical imaginations.
C. The existence of the region of Vinland can never be accurately accounted for in historical terms.
D. The actual location of the region of Vinland remains a matter of debate.

41. It appears as though the author relies most heavily on which of the following sources to develop his argument?

A. Ancient myths and legends
B. Religious records
C. Careful readings of Viking sagas and calculations of sailing times
D. Established historical records

42. Based on the passage, one can conclude that the Viking migration in the New World was most likely driven by:

A. the pursuit of suitable agricultural land.
B. propaganda-based efforts to encourage settlement.
C. further efforts at exploration in general.
D. opposition from established settlements already in the New World.

Passage VII (Questions 43–50)

In many cities, police are accused of inappropriate use of force as a result of the actions they take toward civil rights demonstrators. In many instances, these demonstrators have broken the law. In other cases, the accusations of inappropriate use of force occur in the course of subduing riots or apprehending and searching crime suspects.

However, the policeman's sense of alienation from society results in the development of a distinctive "subculture" or "code" among police officers by which they can live, thus providing a basis for self-respect independent to some degree of civilian attitudes. Whether that subculture or code is based on a commitment to highly professional, austere, and impersonal standards of police conduct or is based on a celebration of the highly personal and particular fraternity of police life (with a tolerant attitude toward misconduct by officers provided that policemen "stand together" against outsiders), depends on many factors. One factor is the quality of police leadership; equally important is the extent to which one police code or another is supported by the political and civil ethos of the community. Maintaining a highly professional police force is probably impossible in a city that does not have a political and civic leadership that attaches a high value to honesty, efficiency, impartiality, and the impersonal application of general rules. By the same token, communities that prefer a politics of personal friendship, of favor giving and receiving, are likely to have police departments that reflect this ethos.

In our large cities where the population is economically and racially heterogeneous and different political styles contend, the morale problem is likely to be particularly critical. Here, the political arrangements are likely to make a commitment to either thorough-going professionalism or police fraternalism both more difficult. It is true that competing pressures on the force will make either choice hard and more necessary. The morale problem will be severe enough to make the development of some code important.

Obviously, there will be many cities, particularly smaller ones, and many occasions within all cities in which the police officer senses little or no hostility and detects few important inconsistencies in goals. Furthermore, in many routine matters, the policeman is likely to be a peace officer rather than a law officer. That is, he is likely to provide assistance rather than to make arrests or enforce laws. And finally, many police administrators argue that a professionalized force will be a respected force, even in the most conflict-laden large city.

The American police officer finds himself today on the grinding edge between the need to maintain his authority on the street and the increased community pressures against that authority. A police force may improve greatly because of professionalization, but if at the same time the popular image and authority of the police officer have deteriorated, the two changes may cancel each other out, producing no net gain in police morale and creating a continuing police problem. In order to maintain morale, the officer may have to rely increasingly on police doctrine, a perhaps exaggerated conception of the rightness of what he is doing, and a contempt for both the criminal and hypocritical noncriminal elements of the population. Under such pressures it is not surprising that many police officers have shown themselves amenable to extremist political positions.

Adapted from Jerome Q. Thomas, "Police Morale, Reform, and Citizen Respect: The Chicago Case" in *The Police*. © 1987 by Waverly Press.

43. The passage most accurately suggests that public attitudes toward police brutality are:

A. completely misguided.
B. perfectly justified.
C. unfairly critical.
D. unfairly exaggerated.

44. According to information in the passage, the average citizen least understands which of the following aspects of police work?

A. The internal politics of police departments
B. The demands placed on police officers by increasing community pressures against his authority
C. The important relationship between politics and police work
D. The consequences of economic and racial heterogeneity in large urban centers

45. When the author notes that "in order to maintain morale, the officer may have to rely increasingly on police doctrine," he is probably referring to an increased reliance on:

A. the strict formalities of police work.
B. his legal status as a law officer.
C. personal as opposed to community efforts at law enforcement.
D. fellow officers as opposed to hypocritical members of the community.

46. The author suggests that policing in smaller urban centers has benefits. How does policing in large urban centers generally compare to policing in smaller urban centers?

A. Large urban areas are more likely to be politically contentious.
B. Large urban areas are more likely to be characterized by conflicting goals.
C. Small urban areas allow the officer to provide assistance rather than enforce laws.
D. Small urban areas are characterized by more professionalized police forces.

47. In the discussion of the "subculture" or "code" among police officers, the passage appears to suggest that:

A. most police officers are essentially forced to "stand together" against outsiders.
B. the existence of police subcultures often leads to a sense of alienation from the rest of society.
C. police subcultures provide an important buffer against critical public attitudes.
D. police subcultures provide for a commitment to highly professional standards of conduct.

48. According to the logic of the passage, it seems reasonable to suggest that the conviction of police officers in the beating of private citizens would work most effectively to:

A. enhance the internal solidarity of police departments.
B. enhance police contempt for the hypocritical noncriminal elements of the population.
C. diminish police commitment to police fraternalism.
D. diminish police commitment to effective police work.

49. Based on the tone of the passage, which statement most accurately captures the author's attitude toward police brutality? Police brutality is:

A. most likely unavoidable in the context of contemporary American society.
B. expected in any large American urban center.
C. most often the result of the public's failure to respect law enforcement officials.
D. an understandable dimension of police work in general.

50. According to information in the passage, a corrupt police department is most often the result of:

A. corruption in local politics.
B. the deterioration of the popular image and authority of police officers in general.
C. exaggerated conceptions of the rightness of what they are doing.
D. corruption in police leadership.

Passage VIII (Questions 51–58)

In a recent essay, Camille Paglia offered a most eloquent overview of the life and death of one of America's most prominent first ladies. In her tribute, Paglia noted that the death of Jacqueline Bouvier Kennedy Onassis on May 19, 1994, was headline news in America and inspired testimonials of love and respect across all divisions of social class and political party. Jackie was the most famous woman in the world in a long period following that of the great stars of Hollywood and preceding our own pop princesses, Diana and Madonna, both currently in semi-eclipse.

In an effort to transcend the purely superficial, Paglia argues that merely as a paragon of high fashion and elegant good taste, Jackie could not have won the position she retained over several decades in millions of people's affections. It was her baptism by gunfire that deified her. Her extraordinary behavior during and after the assassination of her husband has given her a permanent place in history. In the blood-spattered limousine in Dallas, an archetypal *pieta* was forced on Jackie. Cradling the head of the head-of-state in her lap, she became Michelangelo's grieving Madonna, caught between the horror and admiration at the wounded body of her beautiful son. The Catholic Andy Warhol paid tribute to this aspect of her in his Duccio-like checkerboard altarpiece of Jackie as a national *mater dolorosa*.

Jackie's heroism was made possible, submits Paglia, by a neglected element of her famous biography. Everyone knows about her athleticism and cult of fitness, her love of horses from childhood. What we are admiring in her deportment in crisis is dressage, the art of English horsemanship, an aristocratic style that descends from the pre-revolutionary *ancien regime* of the eighteenth century. When people say Jackie is "the closest thing to royalty" American democracy has ever seen, this is what they really mean.

Dressage is described here as a form of radical minimalism, of hierarchical stillness and repose. The rider's signals to the horse are completely invisible. Jackie, masquerading as the perfect adornment, was a master of manipulation and control, not of the psychological realm, where she was at the mercy of adulterous men, but of the physical realm, which she brought to the highest level of refinement. From her renovation of the White House to John F. Kennedy's magnificent state funeral, she simplified, condensed, and reshaped out of her powerful instinct for visual symbolism.

In ancient Greek culture, the image of horse and rider represented the victory of reason in the eternal battle of civilization with anarchy. Horsemanship had a spiritual meaning as the discipline of our animal impulses. As her parents' marriage disintegrated, the very young Jacqueline Bouvier found in the public ritualism of riding a life structure that served her well to the end. She became a custodian of the forms—posting herself at Lyndon Johnson's side as he swore the hurried oath of office on Air Force One, doggedly celebrating her son's third birthday on the day of his father's burial. The educative paradigm in equitation—the patient process of "schooling" colts—was fulfilled in the success with which she reared two unpretentious children who have escaped the whirlwind of self-destructiveness that so often envelops the scions of celebrity.

Thus, for Paglia and the rest of the world, the legacy lives on. What is indelible now is Jackie's fortitude and valor as a survivor of the blood sport of male politics. Some strange law of retribution cut down the wheeler–dealers in Dallas and spared the women at their sides, as in a Greek tragedy such as Euripides's *The Trojan Women*. The stained-suit that Jackie refused to change that day documented the polarities of womanhood: the pastel pink of girlhood and romance and the barbaric red of birth and death.

Adapted from Camille Paglia, *Mona Lisa in Motion: Jacqueline Kennedy Onassis.* © 1994 by Columbia College Publishing.

51. According to the passage, the international status of Jacqueline Bouvier Kennedy Onassis is most accurately attributed to her:

A. sophisticated public image.
B. behavior in the face of adversity.
C. instinct for visual symbolism.
D. ability to manipulate and control.

52. When the authors speaks of "radical minimalism" in the passage, this is meant to describe Jackie Onassis':

A. symbolic importance.
B. creativity.
C. subtlety.
D. refinement.

53. According to the logic of the passage, the author appears to consider the public's image of Jackie Onassis complicated by our failure to:

A. understand her victimization at the hands of adulterous men.
B. understand her rather traumatic childhood.
C. recognize her preoccupation with athleticism and fitness.
D. recognize her training as a young woman.

54. Based on information in the passage, the author appears to be least impressed by Jackie Onassis':

A. political legacy.
B. maternal qualities.
C. love of family.
D. sense of fashion.

55. The parallel comparing Jackie Onassis with "royalty" is used to:

A. illustrate the fascination of Americans with public figures in general.
B. criticize Americans for their continued preoccupation with aristocratic style.
C. draw attention to the sophistication of Jackie Onassis.
D. reexamine the basis for the popularity of Jackie Onassis.

56. Considering the tone of the passage, the author appears to be most critical of which of the following areas?

A. The demands of political life in general
B. The social subordination of women in the United States
C. A poorly informed recognition of the importance of Jackie Onassis
D. The pretentious nature of the children of most public figures

57. When the author of the passage speaks in the end of the "polarities of womanhood," she most probably is talking about:

A. an internal emotional conflict faced by all women.
B. the conflicting demands of marriage, motherhood, and womanhood.
C. the inability to maintain innocence considering the realities of life.
D. the range of experiences faced by all women.

58. The use of artistic imagery in the passage is most effective in demonstrating which of the following observations?

A. The goddess-like qualities of Jackie Onassis
B. The spiritual qualities of Jackie Onassis
C. The religious qualities of Jackie Onassis
D. None of the above

Passage IX (Questions 59–65)

In a rather nontraditional approach to the history of witchcraft in America, Kai Erikson has argued that, historically, there is nothing unique in the fact that Massachusetts Bay should have put people on trial for witchcraft. As the historian Kittredge has pointed out, the whole story should be seen "not as an abnormal outbreak of fanaticism, not as an isolated tragedy, but as a mere incident, a brief and transitory episode in the biography of a terrible, but perfectly natural superstition."

He notes that the idea of witchcraft, of course, is as old as history, but the concept of a malevolent witch who makes a pact with Satan and rejects God did not appear in Europe until the middle of the fourteenth century and does not seem to have made a serious impression on England until well into the sixteenth century. The most comprehensive study of English witchcraft, for example, opens with the year 1558 (the first year of Elizabeth's reign) and gives only passing attention to events occurring before that date.

As such, in many ways witchcraft was brought into England on the same current of change that introduced the Protestant Reformation, and it continued to draw nourishment from the intermittent religious quarrels that broke out during the next century and a half. Perhaps no other form of crime in history has been a better index to social disruption and change, for outbreaks of witchcraft mania have generally taken place in societies that are experiencing a shift of religious focus—societies, we would say, confronting a relocation of boundaries. Throughout the Elizabethan and early Stuart periods, while England was trying to establish a national church and to anchor it in the middle of the violent tides that were sweeping over the rest of Europe, increasing attention was devoted to the subject. Elizabeth herself introduced legislation to clarify the laws dealing with witchcraft, and James I, before becoming King of England, wrote a textbook on demonology, which became a standard reference for years to come.

But it was during the Civil Wars in England that the witchcraft hysteria struck with full force. Many hundreds, probably thousands of witches were burned or hung between the time the Civil Wars began and when Oliver Cromwell emerged as the strong man of the Commonwealth, and no sooner had the mania subsided in England than it broke out all over again in Scotland during the first days of the Restoration. Every important crisis during those years seemed to be punctuated by a rash of witchcraft cases. England did not record its last execution for witchcraft until 1712, but the urgent witch hunts of the Civil War period were never repeated.

With this background in mind, we should not be surprised that New England, too, should experience a moment of panic. It is rather curious that this moment should have arrived so late in the century.

The witchcraft hysteria occupied but a brief moment in the history of the Bay. The first actors to take part in it were a group of excited girls and a few of the less savory figures who drifted around the edges of the community. But the speed with which the other people of the Bay gathered to witness the encounter and accept an active role in it, not to mention the quality of the other persons who were eventually drawn into this vortex of activity, serves as an indicator of the gravity of the issues involved. For a few years, at least, the settlers of Massachusetts were alone in the world, bewildered by the loss of their old identity but not yet aware of their new one, and during this fateful interval they tried to discover some image of themselves by listening to a chorus of voices that whispered to them from the depths of an invisible wilderness.

Adapted from Kai T. Erikson, *Wayward Puritans*. © 1996 by K.T. Erikson.

59. The author's assumption that "there is nothing unique" about witchcraft trials in Massachusetts Bay is most accurately based on the fact that:

A. the idea of witchcraft is as old as history.
B. the condemnation of witchcraft was widespread in both the New World and Europe.
C. nowhere did witchcraft make a serious impression until well into the sixteenth century.
D. Massachusetts Bay was experiencing a period of important social change.

60. It is rather curious that witchcraft hysteria should have arrived so late in the century because of:

A. the cessation of witch-hunts much earlier in England.
B. the relative stability of the colony at this point in time.
C. the clarity of the laws dealing with witchcraft at the time.
D. none of the above.

61. Based on the logic presented in the passage, one might reasonably argue which of the following statements?

A. Members of any community can be very easily persuaded to persecute fellow citizens.
B. Newly formed communities must be continuously wary of potential threats to their existence.
C. Communities based on religious principles are highly vulnerable to dissolution.
D. Community identity is an important factor for its continued existence.

62. When the author speaks of the inhabitants of Massachusetts Bay "listening to a chorus of voices that whispered to them from the depths of an invisible wilderness," he is most probably referring to the:

A. irrational fears of the inhabitants.
B. religious superstitions of the inhabitants.
C. desperation of the inhabitants.
D. confusion of the inhabitants.

63. Considering the information in the passage, the connection between the Massachusetts Bay Colony and the Old World is best described as:

A. highly interdependent.
B. virtually nonexistent.
C. extremely precarious.
D. highly dependent.

64. The author's reliance in the passage on the importance of "crisis" is used to support the:

A. instability of political life in general.
B. vulnerability of relatively "young" settlements.
C. adaptability of relatively "young" settlements to political change.
D. responsiveness of communities to threats to identity.

65. Based on the tone of the passage, the attitude toward the Massachusetts Bay Colony is best described as:

A. mildly sympathetic.
B. mildly critical.
C. relatively neutral.
D. relatively supportive.

Solutions to Verbal Reasoning Practice Test 3

PASSAGE I

1. **C** Always use the process of elimination to dismiss unlikely answer choices. Although it is the vaguest of the four choices, only choice C appears reasonable. The passage, in very general terms, serves only to suggest that democracy in America has negative as well as positive consequences. Choice A should be eliminated because the author makes no effort whatsoever to make any national comparisons. Therefore, although Americans may be nervous, we cannot know from this passage whether they are more or less nervous than other nationalities. The same can be said of choice B. Choice D is incorrect because, although technology is cited as important, technology is only subsumed under the more general category of "modern civilization."
2. **A** Choice A is best because the author offers few details about the specific relationship between modern developments and the new "nervousness." As such, technology is assumed to have an impact, but the specifics are not provided. Choices B and C can be eliminated because they attempt to specify the relationship between technology and nervousness. Therefore, in the absence of appropriate details, these choices appear too speculative. Choice D can be eliminated because the author actually makes no effort to discuss a changing political context—only the changing context in which politics were forced to operate.
3. **D** Although rather general, choice D is best because it simply notes the existence of problems in the midst of prosperity in the United States. Also, because the author makes no effort to discuss nervousness in a more contemporary context, the other choices are dangerously speculative. Choice A is also general but appears to make an observation about life in contemporary America and, thus, is inappropriate. The same can be said of choice B. Choice C should be eliminated because it goes even further and speculates a continued problem for future Americans.
4. **B** The statement by the author most clearly suggests that the tensions and fears were occurring in the more "refined" realms of American society. Therefore, the statement appears rather elitist. Clearly, there is a reference to the lessened sense of new tensions within the context of manual labor or agriculture. Choice A should be eliminated because Beard appears clear (despite the lack of details) that the effects of advancing technology were important dimensions of "modern civilization" and were a key source of nervousness. Choice C is incorrect because the effects were only being "more acutely" felt in the more refined realms but were still felt generally as well. Because choices A and C are incorrect, choice D can be logically eliminated.

5. **A** Of all of the statements, only choice A seems to be appropriate. Developments in technology and modern civilization in general appear to force Americans to be relatively unsatisfied with what they have and to consistently want more. This appears to complicate political participation (although we do not know how exactly) because Americans were unprepared for such changes. Choice B can be eliminated because the reference to "back-to-basics" is too vague. This could, in fact, mean a reference to material goods, or a number of other possibilities. Thus, it is sufficiently unclear to warrant consideration in this context. Although choice C may be a true statement, there is no basis for seeing such a decline as being related to any of the dynamics noted in the passage. Choice D suffers from similar problems in that it is unclear as to any possible relationship of contemporary mental illness to the logic of the passage.

6. **D** Despite the "elitist" character of Beard's discussion of nervousness, he notes that it is felt by all—just to varying degrees. Therefore, although a class system may exist (but limited in comparison to European cultures), every American was experiencing the effects of "modern civilization." Choice A may seem appropriate because the author notes the differences in the existence of aristocratic privilege as being different in America. However, there is no need to believe that it was necessarily unique. Choice B is incorrect because the passage notes a significant difference between the more or less refined. Furthermore, although the situation is different from Europe, distinctions remain in class terms. Choice C also may be true, but it would be difficult to see the connection. Thus, choice C is far too removed from this discussion in the passage.

7. **D** Be careful not to overconclude in answering this question. Choice D is the best choice because one cannot tell from the passage whether restlessness was obviously manifested in terms of dissatisfaction, disillusionment, or ineptitude. Thus, one must remain guarded and choose D here. Choices A, B, and C (as noted) all specify some particular manifestation of restlessness that is not obviously supported in the passage.

PASSAGE II

8. **B** Despite the critical tone of the passage, the author does not appear to suggest that Madonna is without talent. He appears most accurately to suggest that she is more "a genius at getting attention." Choice A may seem appropriate, but Sobran does note that Madonna is indeed somewhat talented (particularly in terms of marketing herself). Choice C also seems acceptable but appears to overstate the woman's significance in terms of creative talent in general. Choice D can be eliminated because the author makes no real effort to argue that Madonna "redirect" her efforts. In fact, it is not even clear that such talents

exist in sufficient quality and quantity to make her more of a successful mainstream entertainer.

9. **C** Despite his criticisms, the author suggests that the combination of religious element with others creates a surreal montage and appears to detract from the "religious" nature of her symbolism, turning it into rather decadent imagery. At first glance, choice A may seem reasonable. However, although critical of Madonna, the author does not appear to go as far as to suggest heresy. The same can be said of choice B in terms of speculation. Choice D can be eliminated because it goes even further and psychoanalyzes Madonna. Although the author genuinely might like to suggest this, he does not.

10. **B** As the author notes, Madonna makes empty efforts to proclaim the importance of her privacy in light of concerted efforts to maintain an extremely public profile. As such, it appears rather odd when she suggests we do not genuinely know her. In the passage, the author suggests that Madonna seemingly fears being too private. Choice A is in complete contradiction to the logic of the passage because the author argues that Madonna is indeed a genius at getting attention. Choice C appears to have little to do with the actual question being asked and is irrelevant. Choice D can be eliminated because there is no basis for assuming that Madonna necessarily "bares all."

11. **B** Considering the author's tone in the passage, it seems safest to assume that image takes priority over actual talent for many entertainers. In a sense, the author implies that Americans are highly receptive to effective publicity tactics and value them often at the expense of ability. This makes choice B better than choice D. Although the author is clearly critical of American sensibilities, there is no real effort here to suggest that Americans are "unsophisticated." Thus, choice A should be avoided. Choice C suggests an almost unwitting acceptance of showmanship, and the author does imply that Americans are receptive to such tactics rather than being distracted by them. However, this choice does not best answer the question being asked.

12. **D** The passage is used to argue that great success can be achieved by mediocre entertainers. In the author's citation of those who support Madonna, the point appears to be that the "politics" of Madonna's self-presentation have superseded the merits of her genuine creative talents. Choice A is a poor choice because the support for Madonna appears firmly based on her "progressiveness" in general. Choice B is incorrect because no mention is made of a denial of feminism at all in terms of the entertainer. In fact, Paglia (noted as a supporter) is referred to as an "antifeminist feminist" (i.e., not denying feminism but seemingly revising it). Choice C is easily eliminated. Madonna is, in fact, being applauded for her manipulation of sexuality.

13. **D** The author speculates that Madonna's heritage is one quite possibly reflective of a long history of "self-absorbed, uninteresting people." Of course, this may not be accurate. However, the author clearly implies such a conclusion. Although choice A seems reasonable, the

examples offered are limited to a specific reference to particular entertainers and are not fairly generalizable to the industry itself. Choice B is inappropriate because rather than a distinction, the examples are offered as bases of similarity. Choice C should also be eliminated because no effort is made in the passage to speak of the American population from this particular line of argument—although parallels are clearly made elsewhere.

14. **C** Rather than overtly criticizing the press, the best the author does is to suggest that the media have seized upon Madonna's popularity and capitalized on it. Although he may be critical of the press, he does not offer any clear judgment in these terms. Based on the logic presented above, it would be unreasonable to pass judgment on the media on behalf of Sobran. Thus, choices A, B, and D should be eliminated.

15. **A** The passage makes it clear that Madonna is sexually liberated. Choice B should be eliminated because a main point of the passage is that Madonna is a calculating individual, clearly aware of what she is doing. Choice C is incorrect because it also is contradicted by the passage. Choice D may be a correct statement; however, in terms of the calculating nature of the entertainer and the tone of the passage, it seems less convincing than choice A.

PASSAGE III

16. **C** Based on information in the passage, it should be concluded that subjectivity is most "dangerous" for the author to the extent that it can compromise the integrity of one's work—particularly if overt efforts are not made to overcome it. Clearly, subjectivity is an aspect of any inquiry. However, it must be carefully guarded to ensure that one's work makes an important and significant contribution. Choice A should be eliminated because such a suggestion is clearly impossible. The point is that subjective decisions are made; but in the conveyance of scientific findings, it is the objective exchange that allows others to appropriately evaluate those findings. Choice B may be a correct statement but certainly is not implied by the author. In fact, major advances are clearly evident based on appropriate research and presentation. Choice D may also be true, but there is no evidence here that it affects the actual exchange of information, just its final evaluation and integrity.

17. **A** Choice A is the best choice based on the general argument of the passage and the potential for success based on clarity. Clarity again provides for the appropriate bases on which others may evaluate the quality and contribution of one's work. Choice B should be eliminated simply because the author makes no effort to argue the pervasiveness of poor expression but rather how it may affect scientific writing. Choice D can be eliminated for similar reasons. Choice C may be a

true statement, but this is a secondary consideration. The passage suggests that good research and clarity bring respect from peers.

18. **B** As the author notes, a critical sense allows one to reexamine the details of one's work and thus contributes to further success in future endeavors. Therefore, rather than simply being complementary, a critical sense and the quality of one's work reaffirm and apparently promote one another. Choice A seems reasonable but, as noted, appears to understate the importance of the relationship the author wishes to imply. Choices C and D are incorrect because they violate central points made in the passage.

19. **C** Considering the author's central focus on the importance of writing, choice C is the best choice. Although other choices may reflect secondary themes of the passage, the reciprocal nature of research and writing is best reflected in choice C. Choice A should be eliminated simply because of its discouraging tone. Although the author wishes to note that poor work may be masked by certain forms of presentation, he does not suggest that scientists should necessarily reflect on personal limitations. Choice B is a true statement; however, it appears to understate the objective of the passage in terms of how good writing makes positive contributions to one's success. Choice D can be eliminated because it only glosses over the key elements of the discussion and appears relatively superficial.

20. **D** As the author notes, scientific jargon very often "alerts" the supervisor to a low level of creativity and possibly "gaping holes" in the research. As such, scientific jargon is used to mask poor scientific research. Choice A may sometimes, but not always, be true. The use of scientific jargon may indicate the esoteric character of research, but the author makes no effort to suggest that it should be abandoned altogether. Choice B can be eliminated because it overconcludes from the passage. Although technical language is common, it does not mean that it is too commonplace. Choice C is incorrect because it is both unsupported and, in part, contradicted by the message in the passage. Choice D best captures the author's attitude.

21. **B** The central objective of the author is to emphasize the importance of a sound, written record of the process and results of research. With this central objective in mind, it should be clear that choice B is best. Choice A should be eliminated because, although the author assumes that good scientists demonstrate such abilities, these are not necessarily a guarantee that work will be presented in the most effective manner. Choice C is easily eliminated, as the author makes no reference in the passage to recording the "merits" of one's research. In fact, the merits of research are determined by those who are able to evaluate that research from a clear and concise presentation itself. Because choices A and C are incorrect, choice D is logically eliminated.

PASSAGE IV

22. **C** The best answer to this question should reaffirm the author's argument that Americans generally have failed to pay sufficient attention to Canadian politics. Thus, historical ambivalence is based most appropriately on a lack of information about Canada. Although Americans may lack knowledge about Canada, the author makes no effort to suggest that they necessarily misunderstand the connection of the two countries. This bit of information allows choice A to be eliminated. Choice B is incorrect because the author does make explicit reference to Canada's historical importance at the international level. Choice D can be eliminated because it implies that Canada is also a political opponent. This is much to the contrary of what the author describes in the passage.

23. **C** In terms of inferring an American "stance" toward Canada, choice C is most appropriate. The author consistently critiques our (American) general lack of interest. No specific "agenda" is implied, other than the fact that a major problem has been that of ambivalence. Choices A, B, and D all imply some specific agenda, which is not stated or implied by the author anywhere in the passage.

24. **D** As the author notes, contemporary discontent in Quebec is largely the result of "the gaping wound of Quebec's disaffection," which appears to be fed (in contemporary terms) by failures in largely economic terms. This is addressed by none of the choices offered. Because the emphasis here is on the "contemporary" discontent in Quebec, although historical experience is important, it appears to have been successfully guarded against at least to some extent. Thus, although Quebec may feel culturally superior, contemporary dissatisfaction appears more appropriately based elsewhere. Choice B should also be eliminated because the author notes that the government has made concerted efforts to recognize the importance and value of francophone culture.

25. **A** In this question, we are asked about "most Canadians." The answer to this question should reflect the country's general experience. Choice A is the best choice because it refers to a national experience. Choice B should be eliminated because the reference to economic failings appears restricted to the province of Quebec alone. Choice C is also inappropriate because it suggests something that is not substantiated by information in the passage. Rather than a lack of commitment by all, the author seems to argue that the populace is relatively skeptical about continuation. Choice D may be a true statement, but it is too speculative and not adequately supported.

26. **C** The most reasonable answer argues the generally precarious nature of nationhood. Although it is true that Canada faces critical problems experienced by many other nations, its particular historical experience has made it difficult to diffuse the potential effects of such problems. In this context, the author appears to argue that nationhood is never

guaranteed and can be compromised in certain situations. Choice A should be eliminated because it fails to capture the general point of the author's introduction and is overly speculative. Choice B appears reasonable; however, it also appears rather secondary to the more important point made by choice A. Choice D may be a true statement, but the author offers no evidence on which to base such an argument.

27. **D** Rather than assuming a general Canadian submission to dissolution, the author accurately suggests that most Canadians are generally skeptical about the prospects for continuation. Note the author's reference to the fact that Canadians "might let their nation sunder by default." Choice A should be eliminated because it implies a more overt acceptance of failure than the author is willing to admit in the passage. Choice B is also inappropriate because it almost suggests a lack of concern or interest altogether. Choice C, at the same time, appears to overstate the national feeling.

28. **C** This question requires the use of inference. Information in the passage seems to suggest that as an international player, Canada is considered relatively noncontroversial. At first glance, choice A seems reasonable. Yet, in terms of the more general relevance for international politics, choice C best captures the author's central point. Although choice B is noted by the author in the passage, it is too specific. The question is a general one with international relevance. Choice B is specific to the United States. Choice D is logically eliminated, as there is one best answer (choice C) to this question.

PASSAGE V

29. **C** As the author notes in the passage, although nomadism has been considered primitive, it does reflect a relatively high level of sophistication and organization historically neglected by analysts. Our failure to clearly recognize the dynamics of nomadic existence appears to have been the greatest contributor to misunderstanding. Choice A should be eliminated because the contrast with settled communities has itself been based on a misunderstanding of nomadism in the first place. As such, the comparison is misinformed from the beginning. Choice B is essentially a reflection of our lack of knowledge and should be eliminated. Choice D is a true statement, but it captures only one aspect of a much more elaborate image of nomadism as offered by the author.

30. **D** The author's reference to Napoleonic military strategy implies that nomad armies were indeed well-suited for battle for a number of reasons. Note the author's reference to the real strength of armies in terms of both size and speed and the particular mobility of nomad forces. Although choice A may seem reasonable, the author more clearly suggests expediency and mobility, rather than sophistication. Choice B is a true statement but is best understood as a result of the larger character of the armies themselves. Choice C is also a true

statement; however, it does not adequately explain the reference to Napoleonic military strategy.

31. **C** The best choice makes explicit reference to the author's emphasis on the constraints of permanent settlements. As the author indicates in paragraph one, the mobility of nomadic communities made pasture "nearly limitless in extent" and "while he could keep moving, his herds could be of great size." Although the author suggests the greater effectiveness of nomadic armies, he does not suggest that settled communities necessarily failed to mount successful military defenses. As such, choice A should be eliminated. Choice B is unsupported by the passage. Choice D appears reasonable but is not the best choice. The wealth of nomadic communities appears tied to mobility, and the author does not reasonably discuss the "potential wealth" of settled communities.

32. **C** The analogy of nomads and locusts is used most effectively to note the adaptability of nomad communities in general. Pay attention to the numerous dynamics cited by the author in terms of the character of the community of isolated individuals, use of immediate resources, and reactions to the exhaustion of such resources. The analogy is multifaceted and is best captured by choice C. Choice A is reasonable but fails to capture the entire point the author wishes to make. Choice B is limited for the same reasons. Choice D should be eliminated for similar reasons but also because it appears to overstate a singular set of crucial forces in the lives of nomads.

33. **A** Where the author discusses intellectual controversies in paragraph four, the key point appears to be that dissensus reflects a more general misunderstanding of nomadism rather than any specific point. Choice B is suggested here; however, although the author notes the disagreement over the importance of climatic changes, he does not suggest that they were, in fact, negligible as such. Choice C is also referenced but is only qualified by the author as having been overly considered by historians in general. Choice D should be eliminated because the author does not suggest that the movement of nomad communities are explained by climate changes.

34. **D** Although the author makes reference in the passage to success and failure, he offers no particular details for either. Therefore, only choice D is appropriate. Choice A should be eliminated because all of the tribes noted by the author appear to have successfully "conquered" settled communities. Therefore, no contrast is offered by this choice. Choice B is also inappropriate in that neither tolerance nor acceptance is necessarily offered as the reason for abandoning nomadism. Choice C is irrelevant here.

35. **C** The best choice should capture one of the most central themes of the passage in general. Although the other choices may seem reasonable, none have the more general relevance than choice C. Choice A should be eliminated because the author never makes any explicit reference to adaptation in terms of changing political conditions. Choice B

seems reasonable considering some important points in the passage; however, its generalization in more contemporary terms appears more limited. Choice D is inappropriate for similar reasons.

PASSAGE VI

36. **D** The central theme of the passage appears to be that there are a number of key points about New World history in general that we know little about. Although these may indeed include information about the Vikings, it is clearly not limited to them. Choice A seems reasonable, but the lack of information about New World history is not limited to the Vikings alone. Choice B should be eliminated because the author notes that the Vikings do not claim to have been the first visitors to the New World. Choice C is unsupported and unreasonable.

37. **B** According to the author, the Vikings are assumed to have arrived in the New World around AD 1000. In his reference to an ancient Latin text, the author notes an earlier trip seemingly made some four centuries before the Vikings. Therefore, the best choice in terms of a "first recorded" visit is around AD 600. Choice A is incorrect because it makes reference to the voyage of a Viking. Choice C suffers the same problem. Choice D should be eliminated because it provides only the author's reference point for most historians.

38. **C** Considering the author's presentation, the best choice is that which notes the author's questioning of what is assumed to be common knowledge about the settlement of the New World. After carefully reading the passage, one should note that the author is skeptical about existing assumptions. Choice A may seem reasonable; however, it appears to overstate the aggressiveness of the author. Again, his tone is best described here as skeptical rather than overtly critical. Choice B should be eliminated because skepticism is not genuinely presented as sarcasm, which would necessarily rely on a more scathing evaluation of existing knowledge. Choice D might seem reasonable because the author appears to "poke fun" at the geographical choices of the Vikings in paragraph three. However, this appears to be an isolated effort and does not really capture the tone of the entire passage.

39. **B** The author discusses the misconception of ocean crossings in the latter part of the second paragraph. He appears compelled by the fact that the difficulty of ocean crossings was somewhat exaggerated. Choice A should be eliminated simply because, despite his discussion of Vinland, the author makes no such assumption. Choice C should also be eliminated because no argument is made in terms of the sophistication of the Vikings. Choice D may be a true statement, but it seems minor and is actually only implied in the passage itself.

40. **D** The author's discussion of Vinland appears to conclude that the actual location continues to be a source of disagreement. Note the author's statement that "various scholars have put Vinland all over the place" and the fact that he makes no effort to resolve the debate. Choice A is incorrect because although the author suggests the possibility of deft propaganda, he does not make a concerted effort to challenge the existence of Vinland altogether. Choice B should also be eliminated because it seems to trivialize the efforts of historians to pinpoint the location and also implies that the region is fictional. Choice C may be true, but it appears rather speculative, considering the information offered in the passage.

41. **A** A careful reading of the passage reveals that the author relies most heavily on "ancient myths and legends" in his discussion. Paragraphs two, four, and five all make reference to the "sagas" of the Vikings. Note that sagas are best defined as prose narratives of history rather than historical records. Choice B should be eliminated because the author makes reference to religious text, and it is a singular example. Choice C can also be eliminated because it refers only to the final discussion of the location of Vinland. Choice D may seem reasonable; however, historical records appear less consequential than the sagas referenced here.

42. **C** Choice C is based on the author's reference in paragraph three to Ericsson's decision to "head west to see what was out there." Thus, continued exploration appears to have been the key factor. Choice A is an unlikely choice because the author makes no effort to discuss the agricultural habits of the Vikings. Choice B may seem reasonable; however, the passing reference to propaganda is clearly not suggested as the reason for the timing of Ericsson's decision to move in the New World. Choice D is suggested in paragraph two but appears to have no real relevance for the migration discussed in paragraph three.

PASSAGE VII

43. **C** The passage suggests that the public has a limited understanding of the complexities of police departments and police work. Therefore, the author seems to imply that the public could be considered unfairly critical in their general attitudes toward the police. Choice A should be eliminated because it clearly overstates the misunderstanding of the public. Although the author is critical, he does not appear to argue that the public is, in fact, misguided. Choice B seems completely contrary to the objective of the passage in that it accepts public attitude and, thus, condemns the police. Choice D is difficult to ascertain from information in the passage and appears overly speculative.

44. **C** Based on the passage, it is clear that one of the author's main points is the importance of politics in police departments. The author makes reference to political leadership, police leadership, and community attitudes. Each of these contributes to the relevance of choice C. Choice

A may be true but appears to be only one dimension of the larger and more complex political context captured by choice C. Choices B and D are not explored as important elements in the public's consideration of the police.

45. **B** The reference to "police doctrine" is defined by the author as "an exaggerated conception of the rightness of what he is doing" in paragraph five. Therefore, this is easily understood as an enhanced reliance on the officer's formal status. Choice A is not the best choice because it is not explicitly connected to the author's discussion of doctrine in the passage. Choice C appears to be in opposition to the discussion of doctrine in that it emphasizes a shift in the actual role and status of the officer. Choice D should be eliminated because it is not discussed in the passage.

46. **B** A central point made in the passage is that large urban centers are often characterized by conflicting goals. This is due to the presence of competing interests. It seems reasonable to suggest that smaller urban areas would experience less of this conflict. Choice A may be true, but politics is considered to be only one dimension of conflict. Note the author's discussion in paragraph three and reference to politics, economics, race, and inconsistent goals. Choices C and D should both be eliminated because they describe policing in small urban areas and do not really offer a comparison to policing in large urban areas.

47. **C** The author's discussion of police subcultures implies that such subcultures are important to the maintenance of police integrity in the face of criticism. Thus, choice C is best because it addresses overt criticism. Note the author's discussion in paragraph two about the importance of being able to survive independent to some degree of public attitudes. Choice A may be true but appears to overstate the extent to which hostility is manifested in police subcultures. The author notes "standing against outsiders," but it is offered as one possibility in terms of how a department may be constituted. Choice B also may be a correct statement, but it overstates the pervasiveness of alienation. Choice D should be eliminated because it also makes an overstatement in the opposite (more positive) direction.

48. **B** Considering the discussion in the final paragraph of the passage, it appears as though the best choice argues an enhanced alienation from the community in general. The conviction of police officers clearly indicates a formal public condemnation of the police. In response, it seems reasonable to suggest that the police would react against what the author notes as "hypocrisy" in the general community. Choice A may be true but is more implied and less direct than choice B. Choices C and D are unsupported by the passage.

49. **D** Although each of these choices may have some validity, only choice D appears to capture the author's more general attitude toward police brutality. The author also makes no effort to make predictions here as well; thus, choices A and B are unlikely answers. Choice C also should be eliminated because such a connection is not established in the passage.

50. **A** The passage argues that the character of police departments is inevitably tied to the larger political and social context in which it is forced to operate. Therefore, corruption in a police department is both directly and indirectly connected by the author to corruption in the larger political environment. Choice B should be eliminated because deterioration is noted but not argued as the basis for internal corruption. In fact, popular images should be thought of here as the results of corrupt conduct in the department. Choice C is inappropriate because such exaggerations are noted as efforts to maintain morale. Choice D can be eliminated because its connection to the larger context appears more consequential in this particular passage.

PASSAGE VIII

51. **B** According to the author, the most important contributor to the international status of Onassis appears to be her "baptism by gunfire," as noted in paragraph two, and her subsequent conduct. This theme is reaffirmed later in the passage. Thus, her conduct in the face of adversity (choice B) is the best choice. Choice A should be eliminated because the image itself is noted by the author as the result of much more substance. Choice C seems reasonable but less important than choice B. Choice D is incorrect because it has a negative connotation, whereas the author takes a far more positive view of manipulation.

52. **C** By definition, "radical minimalism" refers to understatement and simplicity. Thus, choice C or "subtlety" appears most appropriate. Based on the description in the passage, the other choices do not accurately describe radical minimalism.

53. **D** The author notes that "a neglected element of her famous biography" is precisely her expertise in dressage—an important element in her training as a young woman. Choice A is pointed out by the author but is not established as something the public necessarily fails to understand. Choice B has a similar problem. Choice C should be eliminated because the author notes explicitly that everyone seems to know about it.

54. **D** It seems clear that the author's reference to the fashion sense of Onassis is a relatively unimportant aspect of the passage. Although it may demonstrate sophistication, fashion sense is only a reflection of a much more substantial woman. Choices A, B, and C describe qualities with which the author appears to be impressed.

55. **C** Choice C is explicitly connected to the importance of dressage as a source of the sophistication and ultimate legacy of Onassis. The other choices can be logically eliminated for many reasons. Choice A is incorrect because the author makes no effort to comment on the tastes of Americans for public figures in general. Choice B is inappropriate because criticism is also absent from the passage. Choice D may seem reasonable; however, the parallel is certainly not the "basis" for reexamination.

56. **A** According to information in the passage, it seems clear that Onassis is being applauded for her demonstrations of refinement and sophistication in the face of highly publicized adversity. The author appears to be making a more general comment on the demands of public life. Although the author makes reference to "adulterous men," it is unreasonable to assume that this is the central criticism of the passage. Thus, choice B may be implied but seems overstated. Choice C is clearly inappropriate because the author notes the very obvious public importance of Onassis as a reality. Choice D is implied but is certainly a secondary point.

57. **C** The author's final reference to polarities seems to suggest that "girlhood and romance" reflect a safety and innocence that must eventually confront the more vicious realities of such things as death. Choice C seems to be the best choice in that it captures a rather stark contrast. Choice A should be eliminated because the author makes no real reference to the internal emotional conflicts of women. Choice B may seem reasonable; however, it fails to capture the imagery offered at the end of the passage. Choice D also seems to understate the contrast offered by the author.

58. **A** The use of religious imagery in the passage is best described as an effort to (as the author notes) "deify" Onassis. As such, her "baptism by gunfire" opens the door to the recreation of the woman as a "goddess" or semireligious figure and seemingly elevates her above others. Choices B and C should be eliminated because the author makes no real reference to either the spiritual or religious qualities of Onassis herself—only the consequences of her experiences for her public image. Choice D can be logically eliminated.

Passage IX

59. **D** The best choice should demonstrate the relevance of the author's parallel of the Bay Colony and the European experience. The reference to changing social conditions is most appropriate. Choice A is a correct statement; however, it appears secondary in terms of the details of the author's presentation. Choice B suffers from similar problems. Choice C should be eliminated because it has no real connection to the question.

60. **D** The passage provides no information to explain why witchcraft hysteria arrived so late in the century. The author's curiosity about the late arrival of witchcraft is noted; however, the passage provides no detailed explanation. Choices A, B, and C all make some effort to establish why the author suggests that the late arrival is curious. Once again, there is no information in the passage to substantiate any of these observations.

61. **D** The central point of the author is that the witch hunts somehow contributed to the discovery of "some image of themselves," and a central emphasis is placed on the importance of community identity. Choice A should be eliminated because the author makes no real effort to argue that people are necessarily easily "persuaded" to persecute others, although individuals were certainly persecuted as witches. Choice B suggests a more overt defensive stance for all communities and fails to address the specifics of this particular analysis. Choice C unfairly generalizes religious communities and appears speculative.

62. **C** Information in the passage leads us to believe that the inhabitants of the colony were experiencing a sense of desperation in terms of community and identity. Note again the author's discussion in the final paragraph referring to attempts to "discover" some image of themselves. Choice A is inappropriate because it suggests irrationality, whereas there is a decided rationality (according to the author) behind these final desperate efforts. Choice B should be eliminated because the author makes no such reference. Choice D is implied, but it understates the actual effort to deal with bewilderment.

63. **D** The author's discussion of Massachusetts and the Old World best demonstrates a dependence of the new on the old. Clearly, developments in Europe had an impact on the colony; however, there is no evidence that activities in the colony had any direct impact on the Old World. Choice A should be eliminated because interdependence suggests effects flowing in both directions, and this is not clear from the passage. Choice B is inappropriate because the author clearly notes the relationship of Old World developments and the colony. Choice C may be true, but the passage offers no information to substantiate it.

64. **D** The central theme of the passage is that witch-hunts were somehow integral to efforts to maintain or reestablish stability in the face of disruption, change, and instability. Choice D best captures a central objective of the passage. Choice A seems reasonable but appears vague and certainly fails to effectively and fully capture the author's point. Choices B and C fail to address the key element of crisis.

65. **A** Considering the author's presentation of information about a rather controversial and potentially damaging historic experience, the tone of the passage is best described as mildly sympathetic. The author makes no real or explicit effort to morally evaluate what happened. However, in the attempt to "understand" what happened, the passage appears rather defensive of the experience of the colony. In fact, the

author tries to make complete sense of an experience that others might regard as irrational or frenzied. Choice B is incorrect because there is no evidence that the author is critical of the colony. Choice C should be eliminated because there does appear to be an effort to justify the witch hunts, considering the constraints being faced by colonists. Choice D is a poor choice because the term "supportive" fails to capture the point or attitude of the author.

Interpreting Scores on the Verbal Reasoning Practice Tests

The distribution of raw and scaled scores for Verbal Reasoning Practice Tests 1, 2, and 3 in Chapter 11 are estimated from the performance of Columbia Review MCAT students on these exams. **For each Practice Test, count the number of questions that you answered correctly in the allotted time. This is your raw score.** Convert your raw score to a scaled score, using the following tables. The mean scaled score on each test is 8.0. The standard deviation for each test is 2.0. Many medical school admissions committees consider a verbal reasoning score above the mean—i.e., a score of 9 or greater—the minimum score necessary to be competitive for medical school admission. Good luck!

Verbal Reasoning Test 1

Raw Score	Estimated Scaled Score	Average Estimated Percentile Rank
64–65	14–15	99+
62–63	13	98–99
60–61	12	97
56–59	11	88–96
51–55	10	74–87
46–50	9	58–73
42–45	8	42–57
39–41	7	31–41
34–38	6	18–30
31–33	5	11–17
< 31	1–4	0–10

Verbal Reasoning Test 2

Raw Score	Estimated Scaled Score	Average Estimated Percentile Rank
63–65	14–15	99+
61–62	13	98–99
58–60	12	97
53–57	11	88–96
48–52	10	74–87
44–47	9	58–73
40–43	8	42–57
37–39	7	31–41
32–36	6	18–30
29–31	5	11–17
< 29	1–4	0–10

Verbal Reasoning Test 3

Raw Score	Estimated Scaled Score	Average Estimated Percentile Rank
63–65	14–15	99+
61–62	13	98–99
58–60	12	97
53–57	11	88–96
48–52	10	74–87
44–47	9	58–73
40–43	8	42–57
37–39	7	31–41
32–36	6	18–30
28–31	5	11–17
< 28	1–4	0–10

Verbal Reasoning Powerbuilder

Reading Speed Goal Sheet

Practice Passages	*Reading Speed (Words Per Minute)*
MCAT Passage **I** (Chapter 3)	______________________
MCAT Passage **II** (Chapter 3)	______________________
MCAT Passage **III** (Chapter 3)	______________________
MCAT Passage **IV** (Chapter 4)	______________________
MCAT Passage **V** (Chapter 5)	______________________
MCAT Passage **VI** (Chapter 6)	______________________
MCAT Passage **VII** (Chapter 8)	______________________
MCAT Passage **VIII** (Chapter 9)	______________________
Practice Verbal Reasoning Passages in Chapter 10 *(Average Speed per Passage)*	______________________

APPENDIX

MCAT Verbal Reasoning Vocabulary Development Program

This appendix is designed for students who wish to improve their vocabulary or have an English as a second language (ESL) background. If you do not know whether your verbal skills are a strength or weakness, a good way to find out is to try a Verbal Reasoning test. If you are scoring well above average, you are in good shape. On the other hand, if your performance is average or below average and the vocabulary words are difficult for you, consider working through this section. Another way to determine if you could benefit from vocabulary development is to look back at your SAT verbal performance. **If you scored under 600 on the SAT verbal section, you may wish to review this section.**

Importance of Word Parts

If you have a limited vocabulary or an ESL background, you can benefit from vocabulary development. You can improve your vocabulary in several ways. First, read as much as you can in the year or two before the MCAT. Reading will improve your speed and comprehension as well as vocabulary. Another great way to improve your vocabulary is to learn common prefixes, suffixes, and word roots. Learning new word parts allows you to define thousands of new words. This may help you on the MCAT Verbal Reasoning section when you do not immediately recognize a word.

The possession of a strong vocabulary is a definite factor in Verbal Reasoning success. Figuring out the meaning of a key word in a reading passage may make the difference in your answering a group of questions correctly. For example, several recent MCAT Verbal Reasoning passages have contained fairly difficult vocabulary words. These words were important key words in the passages. Some ESL students taking the MCAT did not understand those words and, therefore, had difficulty understanding the passages. You can avoid this potential disaster! Your recognition of prefixes, roots, and suffixes can help you determine the meanings of many words. You need to review some extremely useful word parts so you can recognize them quickly and associate their meanings with words already in your vocabulary.

The following word-parts review is divided into three sections: **prefixes, roots,** and **suffixes.** Recall that **prefixes are the first parts of words.** For example, in the word *biannual*, the prefix *bi* means two; *annual* means year. Thus, *biannual* means twice a year. **Roots are recognizable components of words,** generally derived from Latin or Greek. Consider the word *contradict*. This word is made up of two roots. *Contra* means to go against; *dict* means to say or pronounce. Thus, the word *contradict* means to express the opposite of a statement. **Suffixes are word parts added to the end of words,** serving to form a new word. For the word *cardiology,* the suffix *ology* means the study of; *cardi* means heart. Thus, cardiology means the study of the heart.

How to Approach the Study of Word Parts

If you wish to improve your vocabulary and have at least 6 to 12 months before the MCAT, consider spending some time studying this section. Learning word parts takes time and practice. This is not something that you should "cram" several weeks before the MCAT. If your studying is rushed or last minute, your time may be better spent on the Verbal Reasoning practice tests and working on other strategies. If you have planned ahead and have time to improve your vocabulary, try to spend some time every day working on word parts. Consider making **flash cards** to learn the meanings of the word parts. See if you can tackle some new word parts every day. The more word parts you know, the better!

Prefixes (Table A-1)

Table A-1. Prefixes

WORD PART	MEANING	EXAMPLES
a, an	lacking, not, without	amoral, anarchy, amorphous
a	on, in, of, up, to	afoul, afore, afoot, amuse
ab, abs	from, off, away	abnormal, abaft, abdicate, aborigine
ad, ac, af, ag, al, an, ap, as, at	to, toward, very	adept, adduce, acknowledge, attune, applaud
ambi, amphi	around, both	ambivalent, amphitheater
ana	up, back, again	anagram, analogue, analysis
ante, anti	before, previous	antebellum, antediluvian
anti	against, opposing	anticlimax, antifreeze, antipathy
ap, apo	from, away	apocalypse, apothecary
arch, archi	chief, first	archangel, archipelago
be	intensely, to make	bedraggle, besiege, berate
bene	good, well	benediction, benefit
bon	good	bon hommie, bon voyage
by	bear, extra	by-election, byroad, bystander
cata, cat, cath	down, away, by, in accordance with	catalog, catapult, catheter
circum	around, about	circumspect, circumflex
com, co, col, con	with, together, very	copilot, collaborate, concave
contra, counter	against, opposing	contrary, counterclockwise
de	from, down, off, away	descend, devalue, decompose
demi	half	demibastion, demimonde
dia	through, across, apart	diagonal, diagram, diatribe

Table A-1. Prefixes (continued)

WORD PART	MEANING	EXAMPLES
di, dif, dis	away, opposing, separate	dilate, difficult, disability, disarray
e, ef, ex	away, from, out	erase, expose
en, em	in, among, within	enact, employ
epi	on, outside, over, outer	epicenter, epidemic
eu	good, well	euphoria, euthanasia, eulogize
ex	former	ex-senator, ex-boyfriend
exo	outside, outer	exoskeleton, exotic, exosphere
extra, exter, extro	outside, beyond	extracurricular, exterior, extroversion
for	against, away	forbear, forage
fore	before	foresee, foreman, foreshadow
hetero	other, different	heteronomy, heterogeneity
homo, home, homeo, homi	same, similar	homeopathy, homicide, homosphere
hyper	above, beyond, super	hypersensitive, hyperacidity
hyp, hypo	under, down	hypochondria, hypocrisy, hypothesis
in, il, im, ir	in, into; not, opposing	insecure, inconsecutive, implant, irrelevant, incognito
inter	among, between	interject, interceptor, intercede
intro, intra	inwardly, to the inside	intramuscular, introspect
macr, macro	long, large	macronutrient, macroscopic
mal, male	bad, badly	malediction, malady, malignant, maladjusted
met, meta	change of, over, beyond	metamorphosis, metaphrase, metaphysical
micro	small	micronize, microphone, microwave
mid	middle	midland, midsection
mis	amiss, wrong, bad	misanthrope, mishap
multi	many	multifaceted, multilingual, multimedia
neo	new, latest of a period	neoclassical, New-Latin, neolithic

Table A-1. Prefixes (continued)

WORD PART	MEANING	EXAMPLES
non	not	nonessential, nonferrous, nontoxic
ob, oc, of, op	over, against, toward	obese, obtain, occlude, oppress
out	out, beyond	outsmart, outrage, outcast
over	over, too much	overexpose, overkill, override
para, par	beside, from variation	paralegal, parallel, paragraph
per	through, thoroughly	perception, persuasive
peri	around, near	pericardial, periphery
post	after, following	postwar, postoperative, posterior
pre	before	precede, precaution, preamble
pro [Greek]	before, forward	proponent, proceed
pro [Latin]	forward, favoring	procreate, procrastinate
proto	first, relating to	protohistoric, protoplasm
re	again, backward	rebuttal, recluse, recognize
retro	back, backward	retrocede, retroflux, retroversion
se	away, aside, apart	seclude, secrete, segregate, secret
semi	half, partially	semicolon, semiconscious
sub, suc, suf, sug, sum, sup, sus	under, beneath	subliminal, suspect, subscript
super	over, above, extra	supersonic, superficial
syn, sym, syl, sys	together	syndication, synonymous
tele	far, distant	telepathic, telecast, telekinesis
tra, trans	across, beyond	traduce, transcend, transfiguration
ultra	beyond, excessive	ultrasonic, ultraconservative
un	not, opposing	unabridged, unbridled
with	against	withdrawal, withal

Roots (Table A-2)

Table A-2. Roots

WORD PART	MEANING	EXAMPLES
acer	sharp	acerbate, acetic
act	do, impel	activity, actuate
aev, ev	age, era	primeval, medievalism
agr	field	agricultural, agrarian
ali	other	alienate, aliunde
alter, altr	other, change	altercate, alternator
amic, am	love, friend	amiable, amicable
anima	mind, spirit, soul	inanimate, animation
annu, enniu	year	annually, millennium
apt, pet	adjust, fit	adaptive, ineptitude
aqu	water	aquatics, aquanaut, aqueous
arm	arm, weapon	disarmament, armistice
art	skill, art	artistic, artistry
aud	hear	audition, auditorium
aur	gold	aurous, aureole
bel, bell	war	rebellion, belligerence
ben, bene	good, well	benign, benediction
brev	short, brief	breadth, briefing, breviary
cad, cas	fall	casualty, decadence
cand	white, glowing	candor, incandescent
cap, capt, cept	take, seize	capsulate, intercept, capacity
capit	head	capitalism, decapitate
carn	flesh	reincarnation, carnivore
ced, cede, cess	go, yield	precedent, procession, successor
celer	swift	accelerate, decelerate
cent	hundred	centennial, centigrade, centipede
cern, cert	perceive, make certain	certification, discernible
chrom	color	chromolithograph, chromosomal
cid, cis	kill, cut	suicide, incisive
cit	summon, impel	cite, citable
civ	citizen	civil rights, civility

Table A-2. Roots (continued)

WORD PART	MEANING	EXAMPLES
clam [claim]	shout, cry out	disclaim, clamorous
clar	clear	clarity, clarification
claus, clud, clus	close, shut	cluster, exclude, claustral
clin	bend	incline, recline
cogn	know	cognition, cognate
cornu	horn	cornucopia, unicorn
corp	body	corpulence, corpuscle, corporate
crac, crat	rule, power	bureaucracy, aristocratic
cred	belief, trust	incredibility, credulous
cur	to care	security, curate
cycl	circle, wheel	unicycle, cyclist
da, dat	to give	mandate, datable
deb, debt	to owe	debtor, indebted
dec	ten	decimal, decibel
dent	tooth	denture, dentistry
derm	skin	dermatologist, hypodermic
di, diurn	day	diarist, diurnal
dic, dict	say, word	edict, dictation
dign	worth, worthy	dignitary, dignify
doc, doct, dox	teach, prove	doctrine, doctorate, document
domin	to rule	dominion, predominate
du	two	duplicate, duplex
duc, duct	lead	induce, deduction
dur	hard, lasting	duration, endurance
dyn	force, power	dynasty, dynamite
ego	I, self	egoism, egocentric
equ	equal	equidistant, equivalent
erg, urg	work, power	energize, urgency
err	wander, mistake	error, erratic
eu	good, well, beautiful	eulogy, euphemism
ev	time, ago	medieval, longevity
fac, fict, fect, fy	do, make	facsimile, fictionalize, verify
falls, fals	false	fallacy, falsetto, falsity

Table A-2. Roots (continued)

WORD PART	MEANING	EXAMPLES
fer	bear, yield	infer, fermentation
ferv	boil, bubble	fervor, effervescence
fid	belief, faith	fidelity, infidel
fin	end, limit	finite, finalize
firm	strong	infirm, affirmation
flect, flex	bend, twist	circumflex, inflect
flor	flower	floral, floriculture
flu, fluct	flow	fluidity, flush, fluvial
fort	strong	fortified, fortress
frag, fract	break	fraction, fragile, fragmentation
fug	flee	refugee, fugitive
fus	pour	infusion, fusible
gam	mate, marry	bigamist, monogamy
gen	birth, origin, race	genesis, genetics
geo	earth	geopolitics, geologic
gon	corner, angle	pentagonal, diagonally
grad, gress	step, go	gradual, regress
graph, gram	write, writing	telegraphic, anagram, grapheme
grat	please, favor	gratuity, gratification, ingrate
grav	weight, heavy	gravel, gravimeter, gravitate
greg	flock, group	congregation, desegregate
heli, helio	sun	heliotrope, heliostat
hem	blood	hemoglobin, hemophilia
hom, homo	man	hominid, homunculus
hydr	water	hydration, hydraulic
ign	fire	ignition, igneous
integr	whole, unhurt	integration, integral, integrity
ira	anger, rage	irate, irascibility
iso	same, equal	isotopia
it	go	transit, circuitry
itineri	journey, rad, travel	itinerate, itineracy
ject	throw, hurl, cast	eject, conjecture
jud, jur, jus	judge, swear	perjury, judicial, justify

Table A-2. Roots (continued)

WORD PART	MEANING	EXAMPLES
junct	join	junction, conjunctive
labor	work	laborite, collaborative
leg	law	legality, legislature
leg, lig, lect	choose, read	select, eligible, leguminous
lev	light (in weight)	elevation, levitate
liber	free	liberate, liberal
liter	letter	literacy, literature
lith	rock	monolithic, lithograph
loc	place	local, locomotive
log, loqu, locut	speech, study, word	biology, dialogue, loquacity
luc	light	lucidity, luciferous
magn	large	magnanimous, magnify, magnum
mal	bad	malcontent, malign, malice
man, manu	hand	manual, manacle
mar	sea	marine, maritime
mater, matr	mother	maternity, matriarchal
medi	middle	intermediary, intermediate
mega	enlargement, large	megalomaniac, megalith
merg, mers	dip, plunge	immerge, submerge
metr, meter	measure	metrical, thermometer
min	less, little	diminutive, miniature, minimal
mit, miss	send	permission, missionary
mob, mot	move	emotion, motion, mobilize
mon, monit	warn	monitorial, admonishment
mor	custom, behavior	immoral, moralistic, morale
mor, mort	die, death	morgue, mortician, mortify
moron	fool	moron, moronic
morph	form	anthropomorphic, morphology
multi	many	multifarious, multipurpose
mut, mutat	change	mutant, transmute
nat	born	innate, prenatal
nav	ship, sail	navigator, transnavigate
necr	dead	necrobiosis, necromancy

Table A-2. Roots (continued)

WORD PART	MEANING	EXAMPLES
neg	deny, refuse	negativism, neglect, negligence
nihil	nothing	annihilate, nihilism
nom	law, order, rule	autonomous, economical
nomen, nomin	name	nominee, pronominal
nov	new	novelty, novice
ocul	eye	ocular, oculist
omni	all	omnipotence, omniscient
oper	work	operatic, operative
ora	speak, pray	oracular, oratory
orn	decorate	ornamentation, ornate
oss, oste	bone	ossification, osteopath
pan	all, entire	pandemic, Pandora, panoramic
par	equal	parity, parlay
pater, patr	father	paternalism, patrilineal
path	feeling, suffer, disease	apathetic, pathologist, sympathy
ped	foot; child	pedestrian, pedicure, pediatrics
pel, puls	drive	pulse, repellant, compelling
pend, pens	hang, weigh	dependent, suspender
pet	seek	competitor, petitioner
phil	like, love	bibliophile, philanthropist
phot	light	photosynthesis
plex, plic, ply	fold	duplicate, plexiform
port	carry	deportation, portfolio
pose, pon	place, put	postponement, transpose
pot	power	potency, potentate
press	press	compress, depress, impression
prim	first	prima donna, primary, primitive
quer, quir, quis	ask, seek	prerequisite, querist, require
reg, rig, rect	rule, straight, right	rector, regulate, rigidity
rid, ris	laugh	derisive, ridicule
rog	ask	abrogation, interrogation
rupt	break	corrupt, disruptive
sacr	holy	sacred, sacrosanct

Table A-2. Roots (continued)

WORD PART	MEANING	EXAMPLES
sanct	holy	sanctify, sanctuary, sanctimonious
sci	know	scientific, subconscious
scop	seeing, watch	microscopic, telescope
sed, sid, sess	sit, seat	possession, residue, sedate
seg, sect	cut	dissect, segmentation
sent, sens	feel	dissent, sensation
sequ, secut	follow	consequential, sequacious
sol	alone	soliloquy, solitude, soloist
solv, solu, solut	free, loosen	resolution, solve
son	sound	resonance, sonic
soph	wisdom, wise	philosophically, sophisticate
spec, spic, spect	look, see	circumspect, specimen, spectator
spir	breathe	expire, respiration
stab, stat, stit	firm, standing	institution, stability
string, strict	tie, bind tightly	restriction, strictly
struct	build	destruction, reconstruction
suad, suas	advise	dissuasive, persuade
sum, sumpt	take	assumption, consume, resume
tac, tax	arrange	syntactical, tactician
tang, ting, tact	touch	contingency, intangible, tingle
tempor	time	pro tempore, temporal
ten, tin, tain, tent	hold, contain	intent, retainer, retentive
tend, tens, tent	stretch	distend, extension
tenu	thin	tendon, tenuous
term	end	interminability, terminate
terr, ter	land	terrain, territorial
test	witness	contest, testimonial
the	god	atheist, theological
tom	cut	atom, atomic
tort, tors	twist	contort, distortion, torture
tract	draw, pull	extraction, retract
trib	assign	attribution, tribute
trud, trus	thrust	intrude, obtrusive

Table A-2. Roots (continued)

WORD PART	MEANING	EXAMPLES
turb	agitate	turbid
umbr	shade	umbrella
und	wave	undulate
uni	one	unify, unilateral
urb	city	urbanite, urbiculture
urg	work, power	metallurgist
vac	empty	vacuous, evacuation
vad, vas	go	evade, invasion
ven, vent	come	intervene, venture
ver	true	verify, verisimilitude
verb	word	verbatim, verbosity
vert, vers	turn	divert, reverse
verto	turn	introvert
vest	dress	vestment, vestry
via	road, way	deviation, viaduct
vid, vis	see	provident, visualize
vinc, vict	conquer	convince, victorious
vit, viv	life, lively	survival, vital
voc, wok	call, voice, word	provocation, vocalize
vol	wish	benevolence, malevolent
volv, volut	roll, turn	evolution, revolve
zo	animal	zoology, zoomorphism

Table A-2. Roots (continued)

More Roots

WORD PART	MEANING	EXAMPLES
agog	leader	pedagogy, demagogue
anthro	man	misanthropic
arch	ancient, chief	archaeologist, matriarch
astr, aster	star	asterisk, asteroid, astronomy
auto	self	autobiography, autocracy
bibli	book	biblical, bibliography
bio	life	biological, microbiology
chron, chrono	time	anachronistic, synchronicity
cosm	world, order	cosmic, cosmonaut
crypt	hidden	cryptic, cryptogram
culp	fault, blame	culpability, mea culpa
dipsa	thirst	dipsomania, dipsomaniac
gyne	woman	gynecology, misogynist
glotta	tongue	epiglottis, glottal
heli, helio	sun	heliostat, heliotrope
hem	blood	hemoglobin, hemophilia
hydr	water	hydration, hydraulic
hom, homo	man	hominid, homunculus
phobia	fear	acrophobia, claustrophobia
phon	sound	phonetician, stereophonic
poly	many	polyglot, polytechnical
psych	mind	psychotherapy, psychedelic
pyr	fire	pyretic, pyrophobia
somn	sleep	insomniac, somnambulist
soph	wisdom	philosopher, sophistication
techno, techn	craft	technician, technology
therm	heat	thermos, thermostat

Table A-2. Roots (continued)

Number Roots

WORD PART	MEANING	EXAMPLES
uni, mono, sol	one	monosyllabic, solitary, unify
di, bi, du, duo, diplo	two	digress, biannual, duodecimal
tri, ter	three	triathlon, triplicate
quadr, tetra	four	quadrangle, tetrameter
quinque, quint, penta	five	quintillion, quinquennial, pentathlon
sex, hexa	six	sextuple, hexapod
sept, hepta	seven	septet, heptagonal
oct, octa, octo	eight	octagonal, octogenarian
nona, novem, ennea	nine	nonagenarian, novemdecillon
dec, deca	ten	decade, decameter
duodec, dodeca	twelve	dodecagon, duodenum
cent, hecto, hecato	hundred	centavo, hectoliter
milli, kilo	thousand	millipede, kilogram
myria	ten thousand	myriad, myriameter
meg, mega	million	megabuck, megaton
arch, prim, prin, proto	first	archetype, primeval, principality, protagonist
oligo, pauci	few	oligarch, pauper
multi, myria, poly	many	multilevel, polytheist
ambi, amphi	both	ambidextrous, amphibian

Suffixes (Table A-3)

Although many suffixes do have specific meaning, there are several that mainly indicate the part of speech of the words they help form.

Table A-3. Suffixes
Suffixes that form abstract nouns

WORD PART	MEANING	EXAMPLES
ery		flattery, imagery
mony		matrimony
osity	pertaining to	animosity
age	set of, state of	peonage, verbiage
ship	quality of	courtship, leadership
ance, ence		deference, malevolence
ity, ty	quality, condition	disparity, senility
ness		glibness, gregariousness
ation, ition	act of	congregation, recognition
ion		trepidation
al		perusal, renewal
ment		abridgment, belittlement
dom		freedom, officialdom
hood	state of, quality of	knighthood, sisterhood
ism		atheism, minimalism
er	one who, that which	astronomer, examiner
or	one who, person that	creator, agitator
ist	one who, follower of	botanist, pianist, ritualist
eer	one concerned with	auctioneer, profiteer
isn		equestrian, ruffian
ess	female	actress, giantess, duchess
ee	assoc. with, one that performs	goatee, appointee, escapee
ard, art	possessing a quality	braggart, dullard
ant, ent		defendant
arium	place where, place for	aquarium, terrarium
ory, ray	place where	apiary, promontory, dormitory
trix	female who does specific thing	aviatrix

Table A-3. Suffixes (continued)

Noun suffixes with technical meaning

WORD PART	MEANING	EXAMPLES
archy	form of government	anarchy, hierarchy
arch	a ruler of "archy"	matriarch, monarch
ology	the study of something	cardiology, gerontology
ologist	one who studies an "ology"	cardiologist, musicologist
ics	indicates study or branch of knowledge	ascetics, geriatrics
graphy	field of learning, recording system	calligraphy, cocography
graph	something that writes or records	cardiograph, seismograph
meter	instrument for measuring	barometer, speedometer
itis	inflammation	arthritis, neuritis
scope	instrument for looking	microscope, periscope
cide	killing	genocide, regicide
ician	expert	electrician, optician
osis	abnormal or diseased condition	neurosis, psychosis

Suffixes used to form diminutives

[Diminutives indicate smallness in size. Remember, though, they do not necessarily indicate a smaller size of the thing named by the root.]

WORD PART	EXAMPLES
cle	manacle
kin	manikin
let	hamlet
ule	reticule
ate	articulate, commensurate
ize	energize, vocalize
fy	magnify, rectify, verify

Adjective suffixes

WORD PART	MEANING	EXAMPLES
ful	full of; possessing	dutiful, plentiful
ose	full of; possessing	operose, verbose
ous	full of; containing	cacophonous, nefarious
less	without; not having ability to	heartless, senseless
like	like or similar	catlike, warlike

Table A-3. Suffixes (continued)

Adjective suffixes

WORD PART	MEANING	EXAMPLES
able	when forming an adjective from a noun: suited to; inclined toward	seasonable, valuable, viable
able, ible	when forming an adjective from a verb: apt to be; worthy of being	contestable, reprehensible, irascible
escent	growing, becoming	acquiescent, senescent

General suffixes

Unless otherwise defined, the following adjective **suffixes** relate general ideas such as *like, similar to, tending to,* and *compared to.*

WORD PART	MEANING	EXAMPLES
ant, ent, ian	in the position of; the condition of	incumbent, recalcitrant, strident
ative		indicative
ish		dilettantish, squeamish
ive		inactive, placative
ic		chronic, psychic
ical		maniacal, diabolical
al		aboriginal, cerebral, nocturnal
ly	in the manner of; thus	curtly, heavenly
ory		maledictory, respiratory